Oral Medicine in Practice

Oral Medicine in Practice

Philip-John Lamey, DDS, MB, ChB, BSc, BDS, FDS, RCPS, FFD, RCSI
Michael A. O. Lewis, PhD, BDS, FDS, RCPS

*Department of Oral Medicine and Pathology, Glasgow Dental Hospital and School,
378 Sauchiehall Street, Glasgow G2 3JZ*

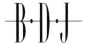

1991

Published by the British Dental Association
64 Wimpole Street, London W1M 8AL

ISBN 0 904588 32 7

Typeset by E. T. Heron (Print) Ltd, Essex

Printed in England by Eyre & Spottiswoode Ltd, London and Margate

Contents

Preface

Over the past twenty years, oral medicine has emerged as a specialty within dentistry and is rapidly gaining increasing importance both nationally and internationally. At the same time, the dominance of surgical procedures within everyday practice has receded and dental surgeons are now more commonly referred to as dental practitioners. While the term oral physician may still be a gleam in the dental profession's eye, there is no doubt that the general dental practitioner is uniquely placed to detect early malignancy, to diagnose and treat common mucosal conditions and orofacial pain, and to discover those tell-tale signs which may be a manifestation of systemic illness.

In view of the need for improved competence in the recognition of diseases involving the oral and para-oral structures, including the salivary glands, I invited Dr Lamey and Dr Lewis to write a highly illustrated series of articles, 'Oral Medicine in Practice', for publication in the *British Dental Journal* in 1989. Now this important series has been extended and published as a BDJ book—the twenty-first title.

'Oral medicine in practice' will prove invaluable to the busy dental practitioner who wishes to increase his/her understanding of oral medicine, to improve recognition of early subtle changes from the normal state and to interpret the implications of these changes and so enhance their standards of patient care. The clinical challenge of oral cancer is mentioned, but the book only gives brief management and treatment regimes as oral cancer was the subject of a recent series of articles in the BDJ, which will be expanded and published separately.

With its coverage of the recognition, treatment and management of many commonly encountered problems in oral medicine, the book will also make essential reading for the mature student embarking on the MGDS and MCCD, and for the undergraduate who, in the new five-year curriculum, will find renewed emphasis on the diagnosis and treatment of oral disease.

Margaret Seward
Editor
September 1991

Acknowledgements

Acknowledgement must be given to Professor D. K. Mason, Department of Oral Medicine and Pathology, University of Glasgow and Professor D. M. Chisholm, Department of Dental Surgery, University of Dundee, for the constant guidance and encouragement they have given to both of us throughout our careers. We are also grateful to Professor D. T. Rees, Baylor College of Dentistry, Dallas and Dr N. B. Simpson, Glasgow Royal Infirmary, for kindly donating slides of HIV infection and dermatological conditions, respectively. In addition, we wish to thank Mr J. B. Davies and the staff at the Department of Dental Illustration, Glasgow Dental Hospital and School, for consistently producing the high-quality photographic material. Thanks are also due to Mrs Linda McGinness, Department of Oral Medicine and Pathology, University of Glasgow, for typing the original manuscript and to Dr Sue Silver, Assistant Editor, *BDJ*, for her help during the preparation of this book. Finally, we are indebted to Mrs Margaret Seward, Editor of the *BDJ*, for her initial invitation to prepare the material contained in this book and her continued enthusiasm during its production.

1

Angular cheilitis

Angular cheilitis is a condition encountered frequently in clinical practice. Detailed assessment and careful management are essential since the presence of a chronic reservoir of infection at other orofacial sites has important therapeutic implications for angular cheilitis. Empirical treatment without adequate investigation will almost certainly result in recurrence of symptoms and failure to detect any underlying systemic disease.

Patients with angular cheilitis frequently present at their general dental practice. Clinical examination combined with an adequate case history will not only permit correct diagnosis, but will also point the practitioner towards appropriate investigation and treatment without the need to seek specialist advice. Close liaison with the patient's general medical practitioner can ensure that thorough haematological and biochemical investigation is achieved. Such an approach to this problem is good practice and advances the link between dentist and doctor as partners in the provision of health care.

Symptoms and signs

The patient's dental status and occupation often give a clue to the cause of the angular cheilitis. As a generalisation, the oral flora of a patient who wears a prosthesis (or orthodontic appliance) is likely to contain *Candida* species, and this is often implicated in the aetiology of the angular cheilitis. In contrast, a dentate individual, with an occupation which requires the wearing of a face mask, such as a theatre sister or hygienist, will often have infection involving *Staphylococcus aureus*. However, the division is not absolute, especially in immunocompromised individuals and those with xerostomia.

Clinically, angular cheilitis may affect one (fig. 1) or both (fig. 2) angles of the mouth. It used to be considered that the clinical appearance of the lesion(s) gave an indication of the likely infective agent, for instance yellow crusting signifying staphylococcal infection; however, this is not correct (fig. 3), since the phage types of *Staph. aureus* isolated from angular cheilitis are rarely those encountered in impetigo, which is typified by yellow crusted skin lesions. Other organisms, in particular haemolytic streptococci, may also be isolated from cases of angular cheilitis, but their significance is unclear.

Although there is no true definition of angular cheilitis, most clinicians regard it as being characterised by inflammatory changes involving redness, soreness and ulceration occurring at one or both angles of the mouth. A classification of the types of clinical changes that occur in angular cheilitis has been proposed, but is not in widespread use. Occasionally, diagnostic difficulty is encountered when recurrent herpes labialis (fig. 4), or erosive lichen planus (fig. 5) affect the angles of the mouth. It is important to take a detailed history of the complaint, its duration, previous treatment and the wearing of any prostheses. A full medical and drug history should also be recorded. Clinical examination should be thorough and clearly must include investigation of the angles themselves, as well as a complete intra-oral examination. The lips need careful inspection and it may be necessary to ask the patient about the presence of lip swelling. Approximately 20% of patients with orofacial

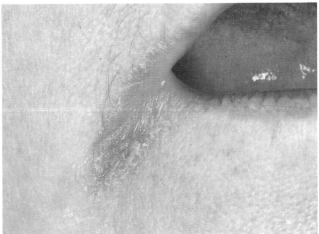
Fig. 1 Unilateral angular cheilitis.

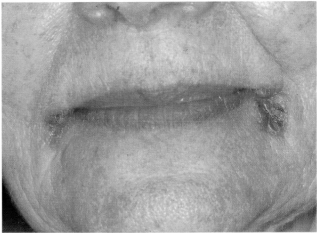
Fig. 2 Bilateral angular cheilitis.

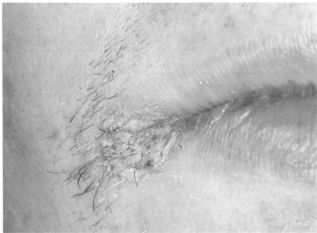
Fig. 3 Yellow crusting does not necessarily make *Staphylococcus* spp. the sole infective agent.

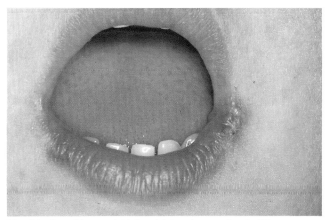

Fig. 4 Lesion of herpes labialis mistaken for angular cheilitis.

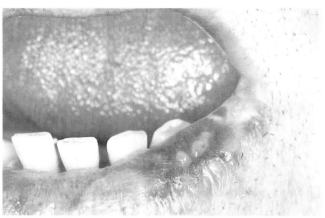

Fig. 5 Erosive lichen planus mistaken for angular cheilitis.

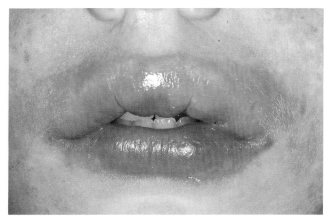

Fig. 6 Orofacial granulomatosis.

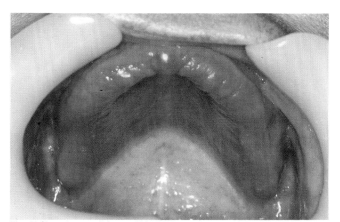

Fig. 7 Chronic atrophic candidosis.

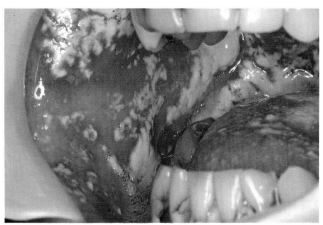

Fig. 8 Acute pseudomembranous candidosis.

granulomatosis suffer from angular cheilitis (fig. 6) for reasons which are not clear but it could be that it is the physical enlargement of the lips owing to lymphoedema which predisposes to infection.

It is crucial to the treatment of angular cheilitis to appreciate that it involves endogenous microorganisms and that these originate from a chronic reservoir of infection. In the case of *Staph. aureus*, the reservoir is usually the anterior nares, since in the UK, 40% of the non-hospital population have nasal carriage of *Staph. aureus*. When *Candida* species are involved (usually *Candida albicans*), the reservoir is always the oral cavity. Figures for the oral carriage of *Candida* vary from 7% to 40% of the general population. When examining the oral cavity, therefore, potential reservoirs of candidal infection should be sought. Chronic atrophic candidosis is frequently present (fig. 7); acute pseudomembranous candidosis (fig. 8), in some cases associated with steroid inhaler therapy (fig. 9), may be noted, as may chronic hyperplastic candidosis (fig. 10) or median rhomboid glossitis (fig. 11). Individuals who are HIV-positive may have a range of intra-oral candidal infections or hairy leukoplakia (fig. 12). It should be noted, however, that even if the oral cavity appears entirely normal, this does *not* exclude the fact that candidal species may still be present in significant numbers.

Investigations and management

A range of microbiological investigations need to be performed for any patient who has angular cheilitis. Swabs (moistened), should be taken from both anterior nares (fig. 13), followed by swabs and smears from both angles and the palate. If a denture or orthodontic appliance is worn, this

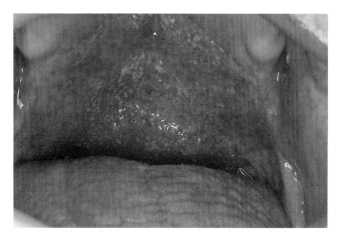

Fig. 9 Candidosis of the soft palate associated with the use of a steroid inhaler.

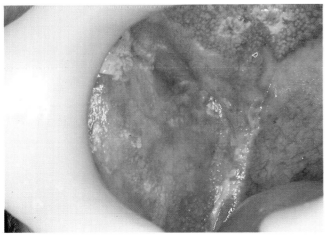

Fig. 10 Chronic hyperplastic candidosis.

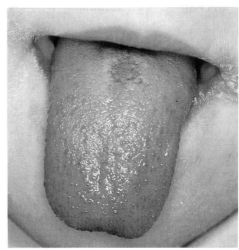

Fig. 11 Median rhomboid glossitis.

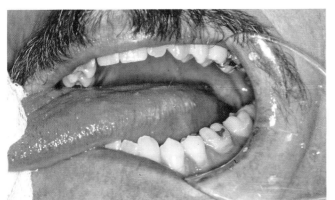

Fig. 12 Hairy leukoplakia.

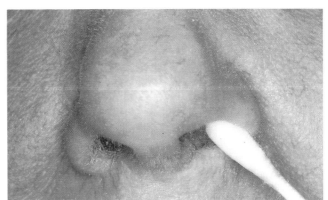

Fig. 13 Swabbing the anterior nares.

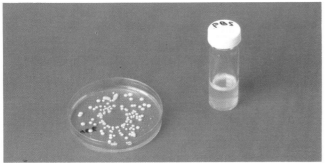

Fig. 14 An oral rinse and spiral plated culture on Sabouraud's medium.

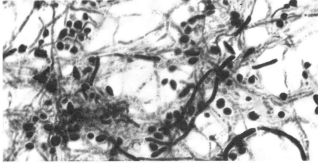

Fig. 15 Smear from angular cheilitis stained by Gram's method.

this should be removed prior to the performance of an oral rinse. In this procedure, 9 ml of phosphate-buffered saline is held in the mouth for one minute, then expectorated back into the bottle (fig. 14). Whilst the patient is doing this, the clinician can take a swab of the fitting surface of the upper denture or appliance, since this site commonly harbours *Candida* species. The samples should be promptly delivered to the laboratory for culture (swabs and rinse) and staining of smears (fig. 15). If immediate transportation is not possible, then overnight storage in a refrigerator is necessary.

Haematological screening, including measurement of haemoglobin, corrected whole blood folate, vitamin B12, ferritin (or iron/total iron binding capacity) and a fasting blood glucose, should be undertaken. In some studies, up to 50% of patients with angular cheilitis have been found to have haematological abnormalities. Clearly such patients require appropriate referral and treatment, to ensure that the patient's ability to fight any infection, including angular

cheilitis, is not compromised. Patients who are suspected of being HIV-positive need referral for counselling and should provide informed consent before screening is undertaken.

The relationship between angular cheilitis and aspects of complete dentures has been the subject of much controversy. Several studies have shown no association between the vertical component of dentures and angular cheilitis. Failure to appreciate that patients may have moderate to high salivary counts of candida without signs of clinical infection has unfortunately clouded this issue.

Treatment

For the purposes of describing treatment, it will be assumed that the patient is HIV-negative, is otherwise well, and that haematological parameters are within the normal range. Treatment will depend primarily on whether the microorganisms involved are either staphylococci or candida, or a mixture of both. If *Staph. aureus* is present, then topical treatment with either fucidic acid or mupirocin cream is appropriate and applications should be continued for 1–2 weeks after clinical resolution. It is important that the patient is given two tubes of the drug of choice, one for exclusive use of the angles and the other for use in the anterior nares. It has been shown by bacteriophage typing of *Staph. aureus*, that the strain present at the angles is the same strain as that found in the nares. The route by which staphylococci gain access to the angles is unclear, but it has been proposed that chronic nose-mouth-finger habits, the prolonged wearing of face masks, jogging, or upper respiratory tract infection are likely to be involved.

If infection is associated with *Candida*, the patient should use an antifungal ointment or cream four times a day for approximately four weeks. In mixed infections, miconazole is appropriate since it has some activity against both *Candida* species and *Staph. aureus*. It is crucial to treat the reservoir of infection within the oral cavity. A nystatin pastille or amphotericin lozenge four times a day for four weeks are the treatments of choice, whether or not intra-oral infection is clinically apparent. If chronic atrophic candidosis is present, then the patient should also apply an antifungal cream to the fitting surfaces of the denture four times a day. It is essential that the patient takes their dentures out at night and soaks them in a dilute hypochlorite solution. A chlorhexidine solution should be used if the dentures have a chrome-cobalt component, since hypochlorite will blacken the metal. In the future, systemic triazole therapy, which has already been proven to be effective in the treatment of oropharyngeal candidosis in HIV patients, may have a potential role in other infections, including angular cheilitis. Recent investigations of angular cheilitis have reported high recurrence rates, but this is inevitable if blood screening is not undertaken, and if reservoirs of infection are not eliminated. Other factors which may need to be considered include orofacial granulomatosis, xerostomia, or allergy (fig. 16). Patients with a dry mouth should be given a saliva substitute (Saliva Orthana, Glandosane or Luborant*), since this will achieve symptomatic relief and aid mechanical cleansing of the mouth.

Failure of treatment

If the steps outlined above have been closely followed, then treatment should be successful. In candidal infections, resistance to either the polyene group (nystatin and amphotericin B), or the imidazoles (miconazole) is not clinically important and any failure of therapy is likely to be due to poor patient compliance and lack of denture hygiene.

*Details can be found at the end of Chapter 8.

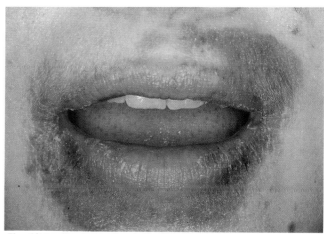

Fig. 16 An allergic reaction to lipstick.

Many patients think that commercial denture cleansers will sterilise dentures, but this is not the case and appropriately diluted hypochlorite solutions (or chlorhexidine) should be used, although some patients dislike the aftertaste.

If lesions persist in patients who report full compliance with therapy, then obviously systemic disease, particularly an immunocompromised state, should be considered. More commonly, however, the presence of a high carbohydrate intake prolongs infection. Many older patients suck hard sweets and this undoubtedly promotes intra-oral candidal growth and, subsequently, angular cheilitis. If patients are unable to reduce their sweet intake, they should use confectionery formulated for diabetics, which has a minimal sugar content. It is also worthwhile asking the patient how much sugar they add to tea or coffee. This can sometimes reveal a surprisingly high intake of carbohydrate.

Drug therapy, including broad spectrum antibiotics, can complicate the management of angular cheilitis. As mentioned, xerostomia needs treatment whether it is due to salivary gland disease (primary or secondary Sjögren's syndrome) or as a result of drug therapy. Through liaison with the patient's medical practitioner, it may be possible to alter drug treatment and achieve some return of salivary function.

Finally, persistent oral candidal infection is a frequent problem in patients who are receiving steroid inhaler therapy. This oropharyngeal candidosis acts as a reservoir of infection, since steroids promote the growth of candida. Reassessment of the patient's respiratory condition by their medical practitioner is helpful, since it may be possible to establish an alternative or reduced steroid drug regime. Alternatively, patients prescribed steroid inhalers should be advised to rinse/gargle with water after inhaler use to minimise the effect of steroid retained in the oropharynx.

2

Oral ulceration

Oral ulceration is probably the oral mucosal condition most frequently seen by general dental and general medical practitioners. It is almost always painful and patients are therefore prompt to seek advice. An important exception to this generalisation is the occurence of oral cancer which is often painless in its early stages. Definitive diagnosis, involving mucosal biopsy, is therefore mandatory for any persistent area of oral ulceration.

There are several initial questions which patients should be asked prior to clinical examination. First, it is important to establish whether the patient has suffered any previous symptoms, since recurrent episodes of ulcers at regular intervals is a characteristic symptom of aphthous stomatitis. The age of the patient is also important, because traumatic ulceration, aphthous stomatitis and acute viral infection are relatively common in children, adolescents and young adults. In contrast to this, the frequency of ulcerative disorders such as erosive lichen planus or pemphigoid increases with age and these disorders tend to affect the middle-aged or elderly. The site of ulceration may also give information which is helpful in diagnosis. For example, aphthous stomatitis does not affect the gingival margin and rarely involves the keratinised mucosa of the dorsum of the tongue or hard palate. If the patient is known to suffer from herpes labialis, then primary herpetic gingivostomatitis can be excluded, although other forms of viral stomatitis would remain a possibility. Other questions which the patient should be asked include: 'Do you have any known allergies?', 'Have you suffered episodes of ulceration affecting your eyes or genitalia?', 'Have you recently started any drug therapy?' and 'Do you generally feel in good health?'

Once the background history to the patient's complaint has been obtained, then a thorough clinical examination should be performed. The main clinical features of the various types of oral ulceration are described below, although further details for some conditions will be given in later chapters.

Traumatic ulceration

Traumatic oral ulceration usually presents as a single ulcer, and patients can often recall an incident which preceded the development of the lesion. The causes of trauma are varied and include injury from a toothbrush (fig. 1), cheek or lip biting (fig. 2), thermal or chemical burns (fig. 3) or damage sustained to the oral soft tissues during an epileptic seizure. In addition, sharp surfaces on teeth restorations, prostheses or dentures, may cause oral ulceration. Rarely, ulceration may be self-induced (fig. 4), although such patients obviously have a psychiatric problem and generally do not admit causing the lesions.

Assuming that the patient appears otherwise well, symptomatic treatment in the form of removal of the suspected traumatic factor and provision of an antiseptic mouthwash, such as chlorhexidine, is all that is required. However, whenever a traumatic aetiology is suspected, the area of ulceration must be seen to heal completely within 7–10 days; biopsy is mandatory for any areas of ulceration which persist beyond this time.

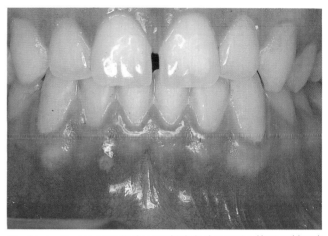

Fig. 1 Irregular ulceration on the attached gingivae caused by toothbrush trauma.

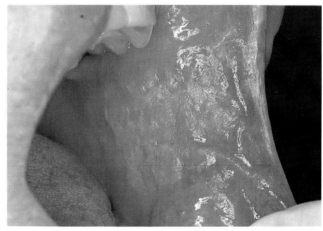

Fig. 2 Characteristic appearance of buccal mucosa in a patient with a cheek biting habit.

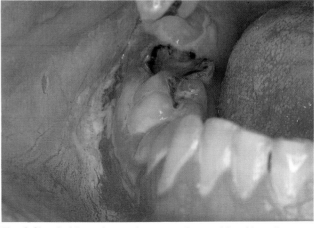

Fig. 3 Chemical burn due to placement of an aspirin tablet adjacent to an abscessed molar tooth.

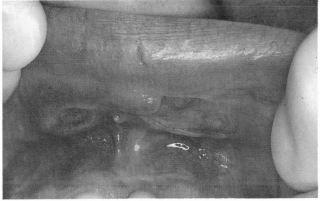

Fig. 4 Self-induced ulceration in a psychologically disturbed patient.

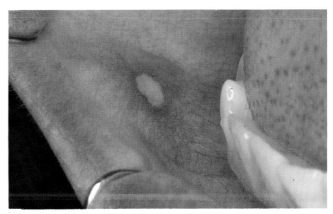

Fig. 5 Minor RAS affecting the buccal mucosa.

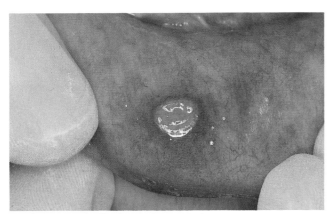

Fig. 6 Minor RAS affecting the lower labial mucosa.

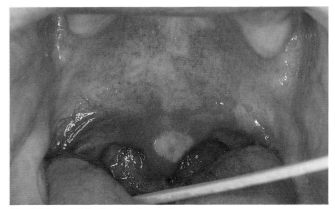

Fig. 7 Major RAS affecting the uvula.

Recurrent aphthous stomatitis (Syn. recurrent oral ulceration)

Approximately one in five of the population in the United Kingdom suffer from recurrent aphthous stomatitis (RAS) at some time in their life. The condition affects males and females equally and is more frequent in the younger age groups. On clinical grounds, three subtypes of RAS are recognised: minor aphthae, major aphthae and herpetiform aphthae. Although these three subtypes share a common feature of recurrent episodes of oral ulceration, there is little evidence that they are variants of the same disease process.

Minor aphthae account for 80% of the cases of RAS and present as ovoid or circular areas of ulceration (2–4 mm diameter) affecting non-keratinised sites in the anterior part of the oral cavity such as buccal mucosa (fig. 5), labial mucosa (fig. 6) or the floor of the mouth. Characteristically, patients with minor aphthae have one to five ulcers at any one time and these heal within 2 weeks. These features are in contrast to patients who suffer major aphthae, which are usually large ulcers (more than 1 cm diameter) affecting the posterior part of the mouth (fig. 7) and keratinised sites. Healing of major aphthae, which accounts for approximately 10% of all cases of RAS, may take several weeks and produce scarring. In recent years, major aphthous stomatitis has been added to the list of oral changes which may indicate the presence of HIV infection (fig. 8). Herpetiform aphthae, which also account for 10% of RAS, are seen more frequently in females and present as multiple small ulcers which coalesce to form larger areas of irregular ulceration (fig. 9). The healing time of herpetiform aphthae is similar to that of minor aphthae.

At the present time, there does not appear to be a single causative factor in RAS, although a number of aetiological and predisposing factors have been described (Table I). There is little doubt that RAS is associated with deficiency states and therefore haematological measurement of haemoglobin, ferritin (or iron/total iron binding capacity), vitamin B12 and corrected whole blood folate should be routine. Estimation of haemoglobin level alone is inadequate, since sideropenia (with normal haemoglobulin and mean corpuscular volume) can be associated with aphthae. Deficiency states are not diseases in themselves, but are a result of either reduced dietary intake, inadequate absorption, failure of utilisation or excessive loss. Therefore, whenever deficiency is detected,

Table I Proposed aetiological factors for recurrent aphthous stomatitis

Factor	Evidence
Deficiency	Occurrence of iron, folic acid, B12 or B-complex deficiency.
Psychological	Increased incidence of RAS in student populations prior to examinations.
Trauma	Development of ulcers at sites following penetration injuries.
Endocrine	Development of RAS in luteal phase of menstrual cycle in some female patients
Allergy	Raised IgE levels and association between certain foodstuffs and development of ulcers.
Smoking	Development of RAS in previously asymptomatic smokers when smoking habit stopped
Hereditary	Increased incidence in children when both parents suffer RAS; also high concordance between twins.
Immunological	Little evidence but some information on abnormal levels of immunoglobulins.

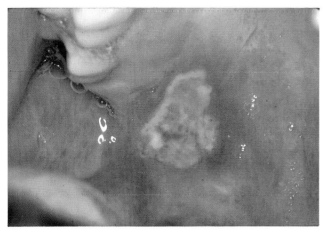

Fig. 8 Major RAS in an HIV-positive patient.

Fig. 9 Herpetiform RAS affecting the upper labial mucosa.

patients should be referred for further investigation, to determine the underlying cause. Sideropenia in women is usually associated with menorrhagia, whereas deficiencies of folic acid or vitamin B12 are suggestive of the presence of either coeliac disease or pernicious anaemia, respectively. In these circumstances, resolution of the ulceration usually occurs following appropriate replacement therapy. There is some evidence to support a role for deficiency of vitamin B1 and vitamin B6 in patients with RAS, although this area requires further study.

Anxiety and stress are likely to be important factors in aphthae, since many sufferers will often associate problems either at work, at home or at college with periods of ulceration. Hypnotherapy or anxiolytic drug therapy can be helpful in the management of patients under these circumstances.

Penetrating injuries of the oral mucosa caused by dental injections or trauma associated with the eating of potato crisps can induce aphthae in susceptible individuals. Females who relate the development of RAS to menstruation usually suffer minor aphthae, which occur in the luteal stage of the menstrual cycle and heal within 7–10 days. Interestingly, hormone replacement therapy in such patients has not been proven to be of benefit and it has therefore been suggested that symptoms may in part be related to premenstrual tension.

Some foodstuffs, in particular chocolate and preservatives, can also cause RAS. If allergy is suspected, then patch-testing to detect potential allergens, followed by an appropriate exclusion diet, may be clinically beneficial. There would appear to be a relationship between smoking and RAS, since some patients begin to suffer aphthae when they stop smoking. The aetiological basis in these circumstances is not clear, but may involve either a stress element or structural mucosal change due to a reduction in hyperkeratosis of the oral epithelium.

In the absence of haematological abnormality, stress or dietary allergen, the treatment of RAS is symptomatic. Although RAS is a common disorder, there have been surprisingly few adequate (double-blind, cross-over) studies of the efficacy of the many mouthwashes, tablets, rinses or pastes presently used in the treatment of the condition. The following treatment regime for patients suffering from RAS has been suggested. At the first visit, obtain a full history, especially the possibility of allergies, and undertake

haematological investigations. Empirical vitamin B1 (300 mg once daily) and vitamin B6 (50 mg tid) therapy should be prescribed with appropriately reduced doses in children. In addition, patients should be advised on the use of chlorhexidine or benzydamine mouthwash and limit their intake of crisps or carbonated drinks. If symptomatic improvement does not occur after 4 weeks, then topical steroid therapy in the form of either hydrocortisone (2·5 mg pellet) or betamethasone (0·5 mg tablet) allowed to dissolve next to the ulcer or used as a mouthwash three times daily should be instituted.

It is important to remember that care should be exercised when considering the use of steroids in children or patients with hypertension, diabetes or gastric ulceration. However, since the majority of patients suffering from RAS are young and in otherwise good health, these factors are not usually a problem. Interestingly, there appears to be a wide variation between individuals in their response to types of topical steroid therapy. Therefore, if treatment using hydrocortisone does not induce a reduction in symptoms, then a change to betamethasone should be considered. Tetracycline mouthwashes, in the form of a 250 mg capsule dissolved in warm water to be used four times daily for 2 weeks, may also be helpful in some patients, particularly those with major aphthae.

Viral infection

Infection due to *Herpes simplex* virus is a common cause of oral ulceration. This may either involve primary infection, which has a characteristic presentation of widespread oral ulceration (fig. 10), or secondary infection, which can cause small areas of recurrent ulceration (fig. 11), particularly in immunocompromised patients. Ulceration due to *Herpes simplex* virus and *Varicella zoster* virus will be discussed in more detail in chapter 4.

Other viruses which can occasionally produce oral ulceration, particularly in children, are the coxsackie group. A characteristic feature of coxsackie viral infection is the fact that it tends to affect the posterior part of the mouth. If a patient presents with oral ulceration in this region, in addition to cutaneous lesions on extremities, then hand, foot and mouth disease may be suspected. Coxsackie infection rarely produces severe pain or systemic upset and treatment is therefore based on symptomatic relief of oral ulceration using an antiseptic mouthwash.

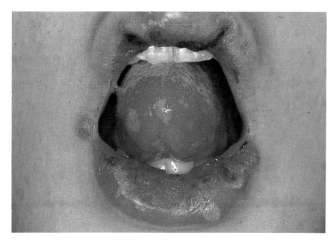

Fig. 10 Primary herpetic gingivostomatitis with typical oral ulceration and blood-crusted lips.

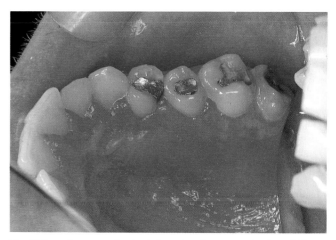

Fig. 11 Irregular areas of palatal ulceration due to reactivation of *Herpes simplex* virus.

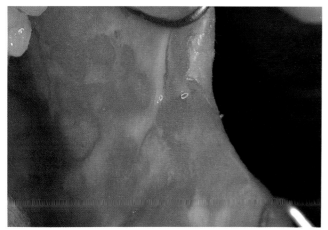

Fig. 12 Extensive oral ulceration of erythema multiforme.

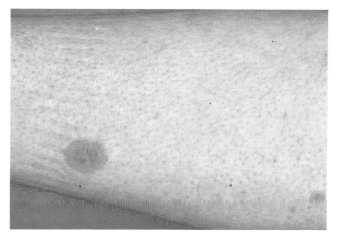

Fig. 13 Cutaneous lesion of erythema multiforme.

Erythema multiforme (Syn. Stevens-Johnson syndrome)

The clinical presentation of erythema multiforme is characterised by the rapid onset of extensive oral ulceration with blood-crusted lips, although cutaneous, ocular and genital lesions may be present. When limited to the oral cavity, the presentation of erythema multiforme (fig. 12) can be identical to that of primary herpetic gingivostomatitis. Both conditions are characterised by the rapid onset of widespread oral ulceration, but if there is a history of herpes labialis, primary herpetic gingivostomatitis can be excluded. In addition, a history of previous, similar episodes of ulceration would also support a diagnosis of erythema multiforme. The differential diagnosis is further simplified if the characteristic cutaneous lesions of erythema multiforme are present (fig. 13). Drugs, particularly sulphonamide-containing antibiotics, preceding viral infection or food sensitivity can induce erythema multiforme in susceptible individuals. It is essential to ensure adequate fluid intake in these circumstances; if there is doubt concerning the patient's ability to maintain fluids, then consultation with his or her medical practitioner is advised since hospitalisation may be required. Otherwise, the treatment of a single episode of erythema multiforme is symptomatic and consists of the use of antiseptic mouthwashes, bed-rest and a soft diet. In patients who suffer recurrent episodes of erythema multiforme, it is worthwhile excluding sensitivity to the benzoate range of perservatives (E210–E219).

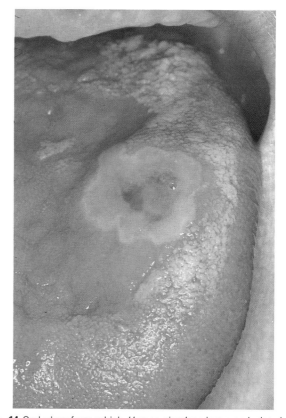

Fig. 14 Oral ulcer from which *Herpes simplex* virus was isolated in a patient with leukaemia.

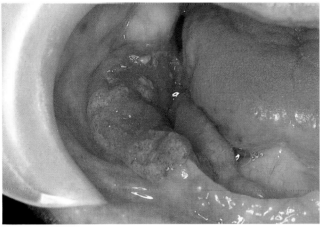

Fig. 15 Advanced squamous cell carcinoma in which bony involvement was evident radiographically.

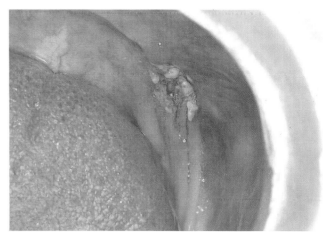

Fig. 16 Early squamous cell carcinoma.

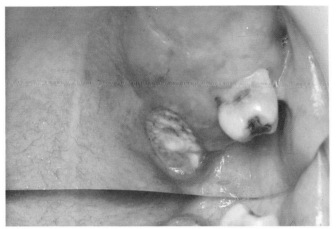

Fig. 17 Maxillary enlargement and ulceration due to non-Hodgkin's lymphoma. (Reprinted by kind permission from *Diagnostic picture tests in dentistry*. London: Wolfe Medical Publications Ltd.)

Myeloproliferative disorders

Oral ulceration may be a feature of either acute or chronic leukaemia. In these individuals, neutropenic ulceration can cause bizarre forms of persistent oral ulceration and infection with *Herpes simplex* virus (fig.14) or Gram-negative organisms occurs frequently.

Syphilis and gonorrhoea

It is rare nowadays to see patients with oral mucosal involvement in syphilis. However, it is a notifiable disease and whenever suspected, referral to a genito-urinary medicine clinic for appropriate blood and microbiological investigations is essential. Oral lesions of gonorrhoea are also uncommon, although infection may cause a pharyngitis in some patients, particularly homosexuals.

Squamous cell carcinoma

Although carcinoma only accounts for 2% of malignant tumours in patients in the UK, it is the most common malignant lesion of the mouth (fig. 15). Since the stage of oral cancer at time of presentation strongly influences the long-term success of treatment, it is essential that any suspected lesions are detected early (fig. 16). This factor emphasises the importance of the 6-monthly dental examination, since this gives the dental surgeon an opportunity to regularly screen the oral mucosa of patients. An example of another neoplasm which may rarely present as oral ulceration is non-Hodgkin's lymphoma (fig. 17). Even less common is oral ulceration due to metastatic spread of tumours from sites distant from the oral cavity. Clearly, it is crucial to biopsy any area of oral ulceration which is suspected of being due to malignancy.

Summary

There are many causes of oral ulceration, but diagnosis should be relatively straightforward following an adequate history, examination and investigation. If the ulceration fails to respond to treatment, or has an unusual appearance, then the presence of an underlying systemic problem such as myeloproliferative disease or HIV infection has to be considered.

3

Burning mouth syndrome

Patients with burning mouth syndrome often report attendance at a number of different practitioners and specialist clinics for treatment of their symptoms, usually with little success. Increasing awareness of the multifactorial aetiology of this common condition and adoption of the multidisciplinary approach outlined here, should lead to successful treatment of the majority of patients.

The term 'burning mouth syndrome' (BMS) is now in widespread use, although, in the past, terms such as 'glossopyrosis', glossodynia', 'stomatopyrosis', 'stomatodynia', and 'oral dysaesthesia' have been used to describe patients complaining of an intra-oral burning sensation. The prevalence of BMS is unknown, but postal surveys have suggested that as many as 14% of post-menopausal women reply positively when asked about oral symptoms of burning. However, this figure should be viewed with caution, since patients were not examined and therefore other causes of a burning sensation in the mouth such as erosive lichen planus or geographic tongue may have been present, rather than BMS.

Signs and symptoms

The signs of BMS are easily described, since the oral mucosa is entirely normal. Indeed, it is not unusual for patients to report that they have been to several doctors or dentists, all of whom have examined the patient's mouth and pronounced it apparently healthy. This in turn may lead the patient to suspect that their complaint is either imaginary or has a psychiatric basis. Interestingly, it is extremely unusual to find a patient suffering from BMS who has ever heard of anyone else with the condition (a factor which heightens cancerphobia and anxiety). BMS affects women much more frequently than men, with a ratio of about 7:1. The mean age of patients is around 60 years, although our youngest patient was a woman of 28 years. At the present time, the condition has never been reported in children.

The site of burning is variable, but most often affects the tongue, followed by the palate/upper alveolus, lips and the lower denture-bearing area (fig. 1). More than one site is usually affected and there is nearly always a bilateral involvement. The distribution of symptomatic areas can give a clue to possible aetiological factors; for example, the involvement of the tip and lateral margin of the tongue suggests a tongue thrusting habit, while symptoms from the dorsum of the tongue suggest tongue posturing, perhaps to hold a non-retentive denture in position.

The nature of the symptoms of BMS tend to fall into three broad categories (Type 1, Type 2 and Type 3). Although in terms of aetiology there are similarities between these subtypes, there is merit in distinguishing between them, since further investigation and indeed prognosis varies with each.

In Type 1 BMS, patients suffer no symptoms on waking, but the burning begins and increases in severity as the day goes on. In Type 2 BMS, the burning is present on waking and persists throughout the day. In both Type 1 and Type 2, symptoms are unremitting and present every day. In contrast

to these findings, patients with Type 3 BMS have symptom-free days and also complain of involvement at unusual sites, such as the floor of the mouth or the throat.

Aetiological factors

Aetiological factors known to be involved in BMS include vitamin B-complex deficiencies, haematological disorders, undiagnosed diabetes, xerostomia, parafunctional habits (such as clenching or tongue thrusting), cancerphobia, anxiety, depression and the climacteric. In a minority of patients, the presence of allergy to materials or foodstuffs may be contributory.

The multifactorial aetiology of BMS lends itself ideally to a team approach to care. Therefore, there are advantages to holding clinics restricted to patients with BMS and staffed by a team of clinicians, including an oral physician, a prosthodontist, a psychiatrist, a clinical psychologist, a dermatologist, and a hypnotherapist. Access to laboratory facilities to process blood samples (full blood count, vitamin B1, B2, B6 and B12, corrected whole blood folate, ferritin, and venous blood plasma glucose) and microbiological tests (oral rinse and swabs) is invaluable.

Although BMS can occur either in dentate or edentulous patients, it is not unusual for patients with dentures to report that the onset of burning coincided with provision of new prostheses. In such circumstances, patients are often convinced that they are allergic to the denture material. However, in practice, allergy to acrylic is rarely proven and

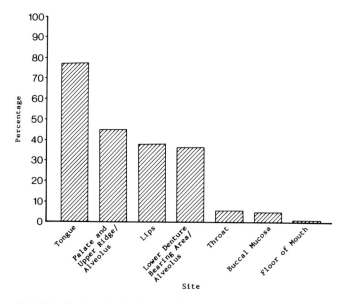

Fig. 1 Distribution of orofacial sites affected by burning mouth syndrome (Reproduced courtesy of *Br Med J*).

it is much more likely that involvement of the dentures is due to lack of freeway space, restricted tongue space or inadequate base extension, with resultant overloading of the denture bearing tissues. The replacement of faulty dentures alone will help about 25% of patients suffering from BMS. Other factors such as haematological deficiency, candidal infection or a degree of xerostomia, which compromise the mucosa, are often also contributory. Clearly, if these problems are not also eliminated, the condition will persist despite the provision of adequately designed dentures.

All patients who present with BMS should be asked to score three aspects on a scale of 0–10. The first question asked is 'How bad is the burning?' The patient is told that a score of 0 would correspond to 'no burning' and a score of 10 would indicate 'intolerable burning'. Such rating is useful in assessing the success of subsequent treatment and is also helpful in terms of determining possible aetiological factors. If a patient has undergone the menopause and all other factors have been considered, the BMS score should be low (approximately 2), since a high score of 9 or 10 cannot be attributable to the climacteric alone. The second question asked concerns the presence of cancerphobia. Patients are asked 'Do you think that the burning is due to cancer in your mouth?' On this occasion, the patient is informed that they should consider a score of 0 to indicate no fear of cancer, whereas a score of 10 equals overwhelming fear. Approximately 20% of BMS patients are cancerphobic and all need reassurance. The final question deals with home circumstances and it is explained that 0 means 'things could not be worse' concerning their family/friends/finance/ housing situation and 10 indicates that 'things could not be better'. The advantage of employing the home circumstances scale is that it overcomes the problem of the patient feeling that the dentist is prying. If a patient gives a score of say 6, then they can be asked a subsequent question: 'What would have to happen to make your score 10/10?' A variety of problems in home circumstances, including marital disharmony, poor housing conditions, illness in relatives and caring for handicapped children have been detected using this approach. This type of questioning greatly increases the likelihood of identifying causes of anxiety or depression, since it permits the patient to voice concern in their own words.

Full psychiatric assessment has a place in the management of patients with BMS, but is not practical for routine use in every patient. However, the general dental practitioner may use the Hospital Anxiety and Depression (HAD)* scale, which can be completed within a few minutes. This scale asks the patient to select one of four answers to 14 apparently innocuous questions. Summation of the scored answers gives a rating which indicates the likelihood of the presence of either anxiety or depression. A score below 8 for anxiety or depression indicates that it is unlikely to be present. A score between 8 to 10 is borderline and a score over 10 indicates likely presence. Use of the scale is also beneficial in patients recording abnormally low scores, since suspicion may be aroused about the truthfulness of their responses.

Management

Management of patients with BMS is straightforward once known aetiological factors have been investigated. Experience has shown that in deficient patients, a course of vitamin B1

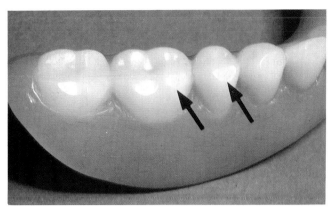

Fig. 2 Lower denture with wear facets on the cusps of molar teeth indicative of a parafunctional habit.

(300 mg once daily) and Vitamin B6 (50 mg tid) for 4 weeks can improve symptoms in the majority of such patients. Indeed, empirical therapy is justified, since at the present time assay of vitamin B1 and B6 is expensive and not often available routinely. Subsequently, detection of haematological abnormalities such as iron, B12 or folic acid deficiency need appropriate further investigation and replacement therapy in conjunction with the patient's medical practitioner. Similarly, patients found to have undiagnosed diabetes mellitus need referral for advice on adequate glycaemic control. In this context, blood investigations are superior to urinalysis for the detection of hyperglycaemia.

It is important to realise that candidal infestation of the oral cavity may be present, although the mucosa may appear clinically normal. An oral rinse technique is the preferred method for detection of candidal infection, since it permits quantification of the candidal load. If the oral rinse yields a significant growth, then antifungal therapy and advice on denture hygiene, if appropriate, should be given.

Reduced salivary gland function can be quantified relatively easily in a hospital setting, although it is unlikely to be practical in general dental practice. Fortunately, however, clinical studies have shown that two questions can be very helpful in determining the difference between the presence of dryness and/or burning. First, ask the patient 'Does your mouth feel dry?', and secondly, 'Are dryness and burning the same thing?' If the answer to these questions is 'yes', then the patient is also likely to report that a drink of water will relieve both dryness and the burning. A variety of saliva substitutes including Saliva Orthana, Glandosane and Luborant are available for patients with xerostomia and reduced salivary gland function (see chapter 8).

Parafunctional habits can be difficult to detect, since patients are often not aware of a tongue thrusting or clenching habit. However, examination of dentures, if worn, can provide a clue, as there may be evidence of abnormal occlusal wear (fig. 2). Approximately 20% of patients with BMS have a parafunctional habit, and it is in this respect that hypnotherapy or tricyclic antidepressants can be useful. It is worth noting, however, that hypnotherapy is contra-indicated in patients who are suffering from depression.

Patients suffering from cancerphobia respond well to reassurance, and in some cases this may be sufficient treatment, provided that other factors involved in BMS have

*Details can be found at the end of the chapter.

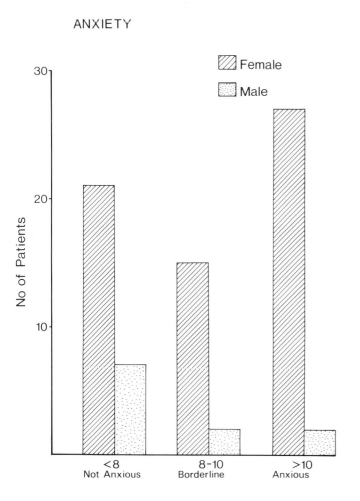

ANXIETY

Fig. 3 Anxiety scores recorded by HAD scale in a group of 74 patients suffering from BMS.

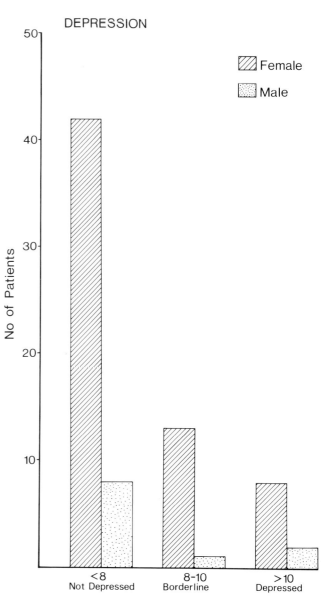

DEPRESSION

Fig. 4 Depression scores recorded by HAD Scale in a group of 74 patients suffering from BMS.

been eliminated. Anxiety is a more important psychological factor in BMS than depression (figs 3 and 4). In these patients, drug therapy, in conjunction with a psychiatric opinion or consultation with the patient's general medical practitioner, can be very effective. Dothiepin (75–150 mg nocte) which has both anxiolytic and antidepressant properties is the drug of choice. Interestingly, dothiepin also appears to be helpful in relieving symptoms in patients with parafunctional habits.

The aetiological factors described above are applicable to all patients with BMS. Two additional factors, food allergy and emotional instability, appear to be particularly important in patients with Type 3 BMS. Suspected allergy to foodstuffs (usually flavourings, colourings or preservatives) or denture base materials should be investigated by a consultant dermatologist with a special interest in patch-testing. A clinical psychologist can be of great value in the management of patients who are suffering emotional instability.

Failure of treatment
The main reason for unsuccessful treatment of BMS appears to be failure to assess all aetiological factors. Adoption of the treatment approach described here in conjunction with the patient's medical practitioner and specialists should allow the dental practitioner to achieve a 70% cure rate. Patients with Type 2 BMS would appear to be the most difficult group to treat. A possible explanation for this is that anxiety arising from internal conscious or unconscious threat is often a major component in these patients. One example of this was the case

of a 70-year-old mother with a 30-year-old son who suffered from Down's syndrome. This lady was frail and no longer felt that she could cope with her home circumstances. Unfortunately, the mental anguish of coming to terms with the inevitable decision to place her son in care was found to be the major cause of her chronic anxiety and subsequent BMS.

Failure of treatment in Type 3 BMS may occur if patients are unable to avoid proven allergens from their environment. Generally, however, once a patient has been found to have an allergy to substances such as sorbic acid, propylene glycol, benzoic acid or cinammon, they endeavour to avoid these allergens. Individuals found to have an allergy to acrylic dentures can benefit from replacement appliances made from either nylon or polycarbonate. Similarly, patients with allergy to chrome or nickel can be given dentures employing gold or nickel-free alloys. An emotionally unstable individual who develops Type 3 BMS is difficult to treat. As with patients with Type 2 BMS, the anxiety component is usually related to conscious or unconscious threat and this often precedes episodes of burning. In one such patient, telephone calls from her daughter who lived overseas, coincided with episodes of BMS, because the daughter had developed breast cancer and the mother was understandably anxious as to the outcome of treatment.

Summary
The dental practitioner, in liaison with medical colleagues, has much to offer patients who suffer BMS. It is important that the history is gained in an unhurried and sympathetic clinical environment, along with subsequent investigations. With such an approach, it is possible to successfully treat the majority of patients with BMS, a condition which at first may seem a very difficult problem to manage.

HAD Scale: Dr R. P. Snaith, Department of Psychiatry, Clinical Sciences Building, St James' University Hospital, Leeds LS9 7TF.

4

Viral infection

Two groups of viruses, herpes and coxsackie, are responsible for the majority of viral conditions which present to the dentist. Mucosal ulceration is the most frequent clinical presentation, although viruses may also be responsible for salivary gland swelling or epithelial hyperplasia. Diagnosis of viral infection is important, since treatment which can alleviate symptoms and reduce the likelihood of spread of infection is available. In addition, the recognition of intra-oral viral infection can have serious implications, since it may be an indication of underlying conditions such as leukaemia, HIV infection or child abuse.

Herpes viruses

The herpes group of viruses includes *Herpes simplex* I, *Herpes simplex* II, *Varicella zoster*, Epstein-Barr virus and cytomegalovirus.

Primary herpetic gingivostomatitis

It is generally accepted that *Herpes simplex* Type I virus is responsible for primary herpetic gingivostomatitis. However, in recent years Type II virus, which was previously associated only with genital lesions, has been increasingly encountered in oral infections. *Herpes simplex* infection is endemic and, by the age of 12, 40% of children in the UK have antibody to *Herpes simplex* virus. The presence of antibody rises to 90% in adults by the age of 60 years. Infection usually occurs during early childhood, although improvements in standard of living in the Western world have been accompanied by a decrease early in the number of cases occurring in life. Infection may produce minimal symptoms or, alternatively, can present with widespread oral ulceration, blood-crusted lips and pyrexia (fig. 1). Patients who acquire primary infection in later adult life seem to suffer symptoms of increased severity, but this may reflect patterns of referral rather than the natural history of the disease.

The lesions of *Herpes simplex* infection develop as intra-epithelial vesicles; however, these soon rupture to leave areas of erosion and ulceration with erythematous margins. Diagnosis of primary *Herpes simplex* infection is usually made from the characteristic clinical appearance, history of contact with patients suffering primary or secondary lesions and lack of skin lesions. Diagnosis can be confirmed either by isolation of the virus from appropriate lesional swabs, or by demonstration of a four-fold or greater rise in antibody titre between symptomatic and convalescent (10–14 days) sera. Owing to the time involved in microbiological and serological investigations, results are not usually available at the time of active infection. Such investigation is useful, however, both in confirming the clinical diagnosis and producing accurate epidemiological data.

Treatment of primary herpetic stomatitis depends on the severity and stage of symptoms at the time of presentation. If a patient has extensive mucosal involvement and presents early, then the use of systemic acyclovir, a specific antiviral agent effective against *Herpes simplex*, should be considered. Systemic acyclovir can be provided either as an elixir (half the adult dose for children under 2 years) or tablets (200 mg, five times daily) for 5 days. The use of acyclovir is not justified in patients with minimal symptoms, or those who present at a later stage. Patients should be advised on the use of an antiseptic mouthwash to reduce secondary bacterial infection of ulcerative lesions. In addition, patients should be actively discouraged from touching lesions, since there is a potential danger of spreading infection to other sites, in particular fingers, nose, eyes or genital areas. Characteristically, symptoms persist for 10–14 days, after which time there is full recovery.

Secondary herpes infection

Approximately 30% of patients who have suffered primary herpetic gingivostomatitis will subsequently suffer from lesions due to reactivation of latent virus in the tissues. The commonest recurrent lesion is herpes labialis (cold sore), which most frequently affects the mucocutaneous junction of the lip (fig. 2). Rarely, lesions may present as areas of intra-oral ulceration, usually affecting the attached gingivae and particularly the mucosa of the hard palate (fig. 3) or buccal mucosa (fig. 4). Factors implicated in virus reactivation include trauma, exposure to sunlight, menstruation or systemic upset. The first sign of viral activity is awareness of a 'prickling' or 'burning' sensation, which is followed within 24 hours by the development of a discrete collection of vesicular swellings. Vesicles soon rupture to produce an area

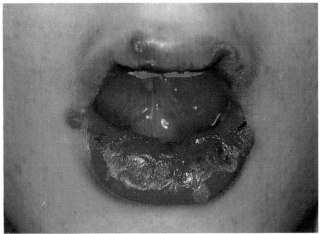

Fig. 1 Extensive oral ulceration of primary herpetic gingivostomatitis.

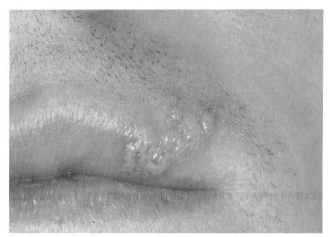

Fig. 2 Early herpes labialis.

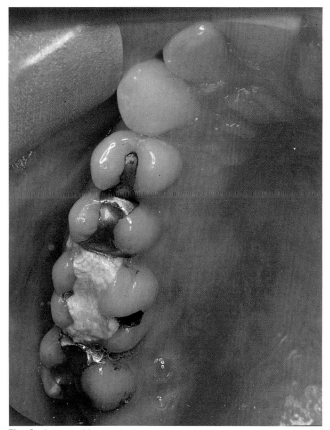

Fig. 3 Intra-oral herpes lesions.

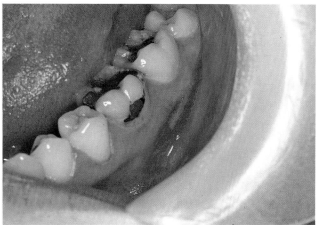

Fig. 4 Recurrent intra-oral herpetic lesion in the buccal sulcus.

of painful erosion (fig. 4), which heals within 7–10 days. In the past, topical idoxuridine in dimethyl sulphoxide was used to treat recurrent herpes infection, but this preparation is non-specific and has been associated with local tissue irritation. Acyclovir has now superceded idoxuridine for *Herpes simplex* infection and can be applied in the form of a cream, three times daily. If topical acyclovir is used, it is essential that treatment is instituted at an early stage if it is to be effective. The use of systemic acyclovir may be justified in patients who suffer frequent recurrences of either herpes labialis or intra-oral lesions. Intra-oral lesions often go unrecognised clinically, but appear to run a similar course to those occurring on the lip and, again, acyclovir has a role in their treatment. Individuals can suffer recurrent intra-oral herpetic infection, but the trigger factors involved are as yet unclear.

Special care should be taken when examining patients with *Herpes simplex* infection, since virus is present in saliva and on the surface of lip or mucosal lesions and can therefore be transmitted to other sites. A particular danger for dental staff is spread of infection into the subcutaneous tissues of the hands through minimal skin abrasions. Cutaneous infection acquired under these circumstances is known as herpetic whitlow and is characterised by the development of a painful vesicular eruption which persists for 2–3 weeks (fig. 5). Prior experience of herpetic infection at other sites such as the lip does not appear to protect against herpetic whitlow. The ability of a dentist with herpetic whitlow to work on patients is severely limited, not only because of pain, but also because of the risk of further spread of infection. Resolution may be slow and it has been suggested that systemic acyclovir (200mg tablets, four times daily for 5 days) is beneficial and may reduce the frequency of recurrent whitlow.

Support for the routine wearing of gloves when treating patients is provided by the fact that most dental surgeons or dental staff who develop herpetic whitlow cannot recall treating a patient with active infection. An explanation for this observation is that a number of patients, particularly children, can secrete *Herpes simplex* virus in saliva for prolonged periods, either following inapparent oral infection or when the oral mucosa appears healthy.

Chickenpox
Primary infection with *Varicella zoster* is responsible for chickenpox, which affects up to 90% of children. Infection is characterised by the development of itchy maculopapular

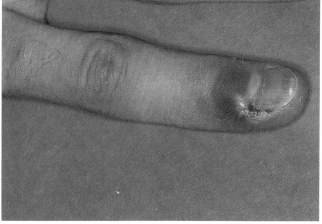

Fig. 5 Herpetic whitlow affecting the finger of a dentist.

lesions on the back, chest and face. Although the condition usually presents on the trunk, the initial site of infection is the upper respiratory tract. Therefore, in some cases, small areas of oral ulceration affecting the palate and fauces may precede the onset of the typical skin rash. However, patients are unlikely to present at the dental surgery with symptoms at this stage and are more likely to attend their general medical practitioner once cutaneous lesions develop. If intra-oral lesions are present, symptomatic treatment with an antiseptic mouthwash is all that is required.

Shingles

Shingles occurs as a result of reactivation of the *Varicella zoster* virus in adult patients and has a tendency to affect nerves. If the maxillary or mandibular division of the trigeminal nerve is involved, then the patient may experience toothache-like pain for several days prior to the onset of more characteristic cutaneous lesions. At an early stage of infection, therefore, the patient may well present at the dental surgery. If clinical examination fails to reveal any dental pathology, then a diagnosis of zoster should be considered, especially in older patients or in younger adults who may be HIV-positive. The temptation to extract teeth with no clinical or radiological pathology in an attempt to relieve the patient of symptoms of pain should therefore be avoided.

The presence of unilateral ulceration (fig. 6) or skin lesions (fig. 7) limited to the area supplied by one division of the trigeminal nerve strongly suggests a diagnosis of zoster. Underlying systemic disease should always be considered as a possible initiating factor in zoster. Treatment is based on the relief of pain with analgesics, and systemic acyclovir therapy. Acyclovir has been found to be effective in the treatment of shingles, since *Varicella zoster* virus has similar replication pathways to that of *Herpes simplex*. However, owing to the reduced activity of the drug against *Varicella zoster*, the therapeutic dose needs to be increased from that used to treat *Herpes simplex* infection. Therefore, for an adult patient, 800 mg five times daily would be routine. Ideally, treatment should be instituted at an early stage, preferably prior to the development of vesicles. At the present time, there is controversy concerning the duration of acyclovir treatment for shingles. A 5-day course has been found to be beneficial, but it has also been suggested that a 10-day course may be more likely to reduce the risk of post-herpetic neuralgia. This factor is important, since the symptoms of post-herpetic neuralgia may be severe and extremely difficult to treat.

Infectious mononucleosis

Infection with Epstein-Barr virus is believed to be responsible for the lymph node enlargement, fever and pharyngeal inflammation seen in patients with infectious mononucleosis. The condition occurs mainly in childhood or early adolescence, and is believed to be predominantly transmitted in saliva during kissing. Oral involvement, which occurs in approximately 30% of patients, includes petechial haemorrhages in the palate and areas of pseudomembranous lesions or ulceration of the mucosa (fig. 8). Rarely, patients may also complain of gingival bleeding, simulating acute ulcerative gingivitis or unilateral pericoronitis. Diagnosis can be confirmed serologically by demonstrating levels of IgM antibody to Epstein-Barr virus, a positive monospot or Paul-

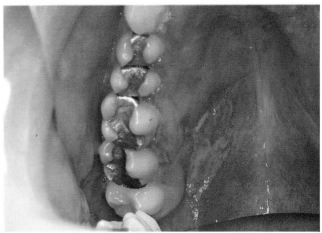
Fig. 6 Unilateral ulceration of the palate due to *Herpes zoster*.

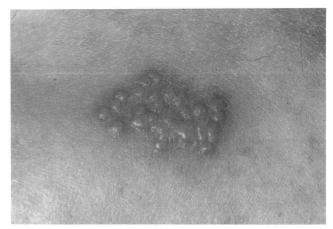
Fig. 7 Cutaneous lesions of *Herpes zoster* infection.

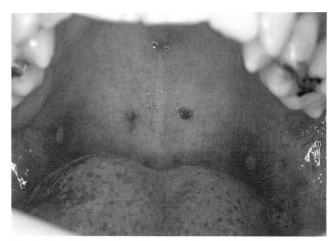
Fig. 8 Palatal ulceration and erythema in a patient with infectious mononucleosis.

Bunnell test. There is no specific treatment for infectious mononucleosis and, fortunately, serious complications are rare. However, infectious mononucleosis has a spectrum of clinical involvement, ranging from minimal systemic upset to serious disease with hepatic or splenic involvement, requiring hospitalisation (fig. 9). Patients should be provided with an antiseptic mouthwash to limit secondary bacterial infection of oral lesions. Amoxycillin or other antibiotics of the penicillin group should be avoided in patients with infectious

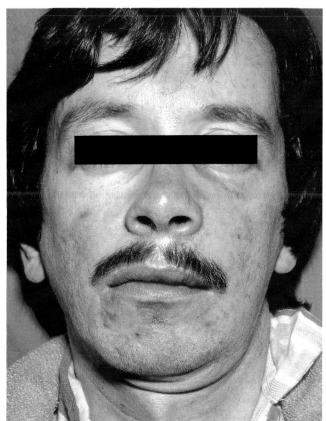

Fig. 9 Patient hospitalised with infectious mononucleosis. This patient developed multiple dental abscesses and thrombocytopenia, which was responsible for the facial purpura.

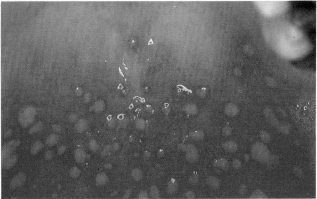

Fig. 10 Herpangina affecting the soft palate.

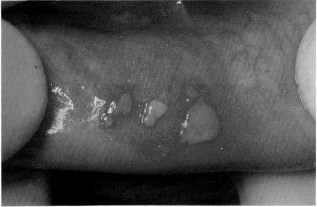

Fig. 11 Oral ulceration in hand, foot and mouth disease.

mononucleosis, since they may predispose to an erythematous skin rash.

Epstein-Barr virus has been implicated in Hodgkin's lymphoma and Burkitt's lymphoma. Burkitt's lymphoma may present as swelling of the jaws, particularly in African children, or as a nasopharyngeal carcinoma, especially in patients of Chinese extraction. More recently, Epstein-Barr virus has also been demonstrated in hairy leukoplakia, the lesion which typically develops on the lateral borders of the tongue in patients immunocompromised by HIV infection or other disease.

Salivary gland inclusion disease
Cytomegalovirus, a relatively harmless virus, can cause a sialadenitis, with salivary gland swelling, known as cytomegalic inclusion disease or salivary gland inclusion disease. However, the condition is uncommon and almost exclusively limited to immunosuppressed patients or the newborn.

Coxsackie viruses
The Coxsackie viruses have a range of clinical manifestations, including oral disease, meningitis, encephalitis or mild febrile illness, and are subdivided into group A and group B. The group A viruses are responsible for two oral conditions, namely herpangina and hand, foot and mouth disease.

Herpangina
Coxsackie types A2, A4, A5, A6 and A8 can produce herpangina, which principally occurs in children. Infection is characterised by sudden onset of pyrexia and sore throat, which is followed within 2 days by oral lesions consisting of multiple vesicles on the soft palate and faucial region (fig. 10). On rare occasions, pain and swelling of the salivary glands may also occur and the clinical presentation may be suggestive of mumps. If clinical doubt exists, definitive serological and animal inoculation tests can be undertaken, but usually only by specialist microbiological laboratories. Symptoms are characteristically mild and no active treatment is required.

Hand, foot and mouth disease
Hand, foot and mouth disease is particularly associated with infection due to Coxsackie type A16, although types A4, A5, A9 and A10 may also be involved. Infection usually occurs in childhood, although adults may occasionally develop the condition. The triad of clinical manifestations consists of multiple shallow oral ulcers (fig 11) accompanied by erythematous macules on the hands (fig. 12) and feet (fig. 13). Diagnosis is straightforward when lesions are present at all three sites, and special investigations are usually unnecessary. If confirmation of diagnosis is required, then serum antibody studies can be undertaken, but, again, usually only in reference laboratories. Treatment is limited to the use of antiseptic mouthwash. The patient or the patient's parents should be warned of the infectivity of the condition.

Paramyxoviruses
Measles
This common infection of childhood has characteristic oral lesions, 'Koplik's spots', which present at an early stage of infection as yellow-white papules with a dark red surround on

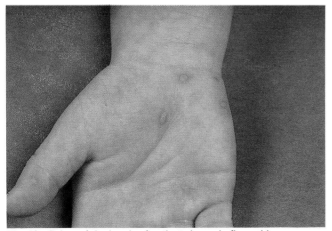

Fig. 12   Palms of the hands of patient shown in figure 11.

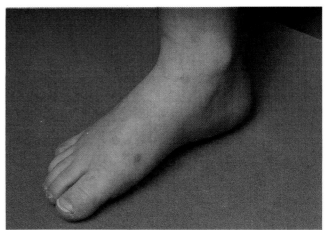

Fig. 13   Macular skin lesions of the feet of patient shown in figure 11 and 12.

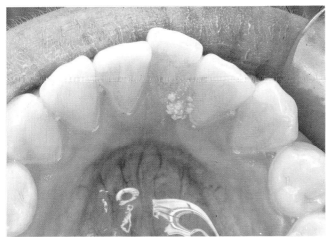

Fig. 14   Squamous cell papilloma affecting the attached gingivae.

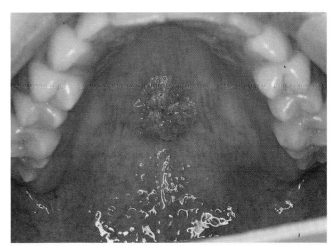

Fig. 15   Condyloma acuminatum of the palatal mucosa in a teenager.

the buccal mucosa. Although it has been claimed that Koplik's spots occur in the majority of patients with measles, in practice they are seldom seen and may, on occasion, have been confused with Fordyce's spots. No specific treatment is required.

Mumps

Mumps is the most common viral infection which affects the salivary glands. Characteristically, the parotid glands are involved, although, on occasion, the submandibular glands may also, or exclusively, be affected. In addition to salivary gland swelling, patients complain of pyrexia, sore throat and pain on eating. Examination may reveal obvious salivary gland swelling, but saliva expressed from the gland(s) remains clear. The incubation period for mumps is 3 weeks and during this time saliva is infectious, which probably accounts for the occurrence of outbreaks within communities. Mumps usually occurs in childhood, but may affect adults, at which time there is a risk of serious complications such as orchitis or oophoritis. Diagnosis can be confirmed routinely by demonstration of antibody to mumps virus. Gland swelling usually resolves within 10–14 days and no specific treatment is indicated.

Papilloma viruses

More than 40 types of human papilloma virus have been isolated. These viruses play a role in a range of diseases, in particular warts, and there is increasing evidence for their possible involvement in oral premalignancy and cancer.

Squamous cell papilloma

Squamous cell papilloma is a common lesion, occurring within the oral cavity (fig. 14). The oral papilloma presents as an exophytic lesion with multiple projections. Patients are often unaware of the presence of a papilloma and the lesions may only be detected as an incidental finding during examination. Treatment is by simple local excision, and inclusion of a wedge of normal tissue at the base of the lesion may reduce the likelihood of recurrence.

Condyloma acuminatum

Condyloma acuminatum is characterised by clusters of sessile papillomatous lesions in the orogenital region. Oral lesions, which may be clinically identical to squamous cell papilloma, can develop as a result of orogenital contact. Once diagnosed histologically, adult patients may admit to the practice of oral sex, either in a heterosexual or homosexual relationship. The development of oral condylomata in children or teenagers (fig. 15) would raise serious concern about the possibility of sexual abuse. In these circumstances, appropriate liaison with the general medical practitioner for the purpose of counselling is essential. Treatment of oral lesions is by simple excision.

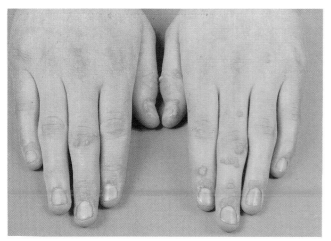

Fig. 16 Cutaneous lesions of verruca vulgaris.

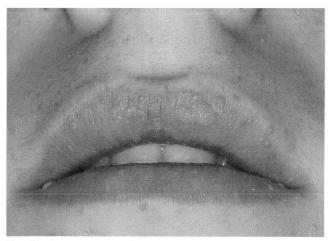

Fig. 17 Peri-oral lesions of verruca vulgaris (same patient as shown in figure 16).

Verruca vulgaris

Verruca vulgaris is a common lesion, which generally affects the skin of children. However, oral lesions, which are clinically and histopathologically indistinguishable from squamous cell papilloma, do develop. The presence of lesions on the fingers is likely to indicate a relationship with the development of any intra-oral or peri-oral lesion (fig. 16 and 17). Treatment is by simple excision or cryosurgery.

Focal epithelial hyperplasia

This otherwise rare disorder is, however, common in certain racial groups, particularly Eskimos and North American Indians. The clinical presentation is characterised by the appearance of multiple papillomatous lesions affecting the oral mucosa. Once diagnosed, no active treatment is required.

Squamous cell carcinoma

Recent research has revealed a possible association between human papillomaviruses and squamous cell carcinoma. This relationship is supported by the development of hairy leukoplakia and oral carcinoma in patients with HIV infection. Papillomaviruses have also been implicated in the development of cervical carcinoma. The role of virus in these lesions is currently being studied.

Summary

Increasing awareness of oral lesions with a viral aetiology and their frequency emphasises the importance of routine wearing of gloves during examination and treatment of patients. Recent advances in antiviral chemotherapy have provided the dental surgeon with effective means of treatment for *Herpes simplex* and *Varicella zoster* infections. However, indiscriminate use of these agents should be avoided, since inappropriate prescribing is both ineffective clinically and costly. Oral viral lesions with an atypical presentation and prolonged duration of viral lesions in the oral cavity may indicate the presence of underlying systemic disease.

5

Orofacial pain

The diagnosis of orofacial pain, particularly of non-dental origin, may present the clinician with a considerable diagnostic problem. Accurate assessment of the history and nature of the pain, combined with good clinical examination, will achieve a correct diagnosis relatively easily. Characteristic features of the symptoms associated with most orofacial pain syndromes are presented in this chapter in table form for quick reference.

Orofacial pain is a common reason for patient attendance at the dental surgery and diagnosis of the cause may initially present the dentist with a problem. However, it is hoped that the approach to pain outlined below will assist the diagnosis of the more common pain syndromes. The nomenclature of certain pain syndromes varies from centre to centre, and in this respect we have elected to use the term temporomandibular joint dysfunction syndrome for the condition others may call facial arthromyalgia and the term periodic migrainous neuralgia for the condition which some may describe as cluster headache.

For practical purposes it is useful to divide orofacial pain into two categories, either dental or non-dental, depending on its origin. Clearly, in the context of this book, it is not possible to consider in detail pain of dental origin, such as that associated with acute dento-alveolar abscess, pericoronitis or dry socket. Fortunately, such conditions are usually well localised and accompanied by obvious characteristic clinical features which readily permit diagnosis (figs 1–3). However, clinical examination in the case of orofacial pain of non-dental origin often reveals no abnormality and therefore diagnosis has to be based on a detailed assessment of the history and nature of the complaint (Table I).

Two key questions 'Is the pain present every day?' and 'Does the pain interfere with sleep?' are helpful at the outset. Following these questions, the patient should be asked to describe the timing and character of the pain during a normal day, from 'the minute they wake up in the morning until they go to bed at night'. Such questioning should reveal how long the pain lasts, whether it is sharp or dull, constant or episodic, or aggravated by certain activities, such as eating or the wearing of dentures. Finally, the patient should be asked to rate the pain on a scale from 0–10, where 0 corresponds to 'no pain' and 10 indicates 'the worst pain experienced'. Such a score will give the clinician a good indication of pain severity and is helpful in monitoring the effect of any subsequent treatment.

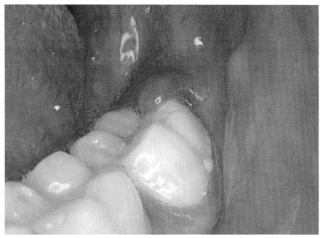

Fig. 2 Pericoronitis affecting a partially erupted lower third molar.

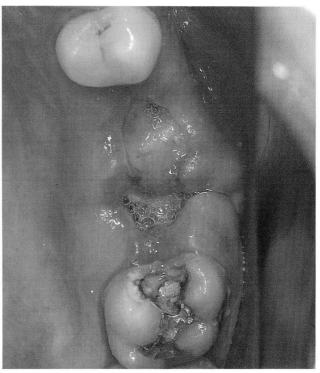

Fig. 1 Acute left side facial swelling associated with a dento-alveolar abscess.

Fig. 3 Dry socket which developed 3 days after tooth extraction.

Timing of pain	Nature of pain	Condition	Comment
Present on waking	Variable	TMJ dysfunction	Associated with nocturnal bruxism or clenching
	Severe and throbbing	Migraine	Clenching may be trigger
	Severe and burning	Burning mouth syndrome (Type 2)	Needs full BMS investigations*
Worse in evening	Variable	TMJ dysfunction	Associated with daytime bruxism or clenching
	Severe and burning	Burning mouth syndrome (Type 1)	Needs full BMS investigations*
Coincides with eating	Diffuse pain or 'tightness'	Salivary gland obstruction	Requires sialography
	Variable	TMJ disease	Structural changes
	Sharp or boring	Giant cell arteritis	Raised ESR
	Severe, shooting, lancinating or piercing	Trigeminal neuralgia	Trigger factors
	Variable and throbbing	Pretrigeminal neuralgia	May mimic pulpitis
	Severe, shooting, lancinating or piercing	Glossopharyngeal neuralgia	Precipitated by swallowing
Disturbs sleep	Severe and episodic	Periodic migrainous neuralgia	Precipitated by alcohol
	Severe and episodic	Paroxysmal facial hemicrania	No facial flushing or running of eyes/nose
Constant	Constant, throbbing or nagging	Atypical facial pain	Exclude organic disease
	Constant and dull	Neoplasms	Requires full investigation
	Burning, gripping, boring or band-like	Psychological disorder	Requires expert assessment
	Severe and throbbing	Acute sinusitis	Increased severity on bending head forwards
Variable	Severe and burning	Burning mouth syndrome (Type 3)	Needs full BMS investigation*
	Burning, gripping, boring or band-like	Psychological disorders	Requires expert assessment
	Variable	Paget's disease	Needs blood and radiographic assessment
	Intense burning	Post-herpetic neuralgia	Hyperaesthesia or paraesthesia
	Variable burning or dull	Ramsey-Hunt syndrome	Vesicles in outer ear

*Details in Chapter 3

Pain of salivary gland origin

Obstruction of a salivary duct is characteristically associated with a complaint of swelling of the affected gland at meal times. When the parotid is involved, patients may complain of unilateral pain in the pre-auricular region on eating. However, since swelling is not always clinically obvious, confusion between salivary obstruction and temporomandibular joint dysfunction (TMJ) syndrome can occur. A complaint of a 'fullness' or 'tightness' in the area of the parotid would support the presence of obstruction rather than TMJ dysfunction.

Submandibular duct obstruction can also present a diagnostic problem for the dentist, although in this situation bimanual palpation should demonstrate an enlarged or tender gland. Confusion with temporomandibular joint dysfunction can occur if the source of any tenderness detected is the medial pterygoid muscle, rather than the submandibular gland.

Sialography is more helpful than radiography in the diagnosis of salivary gland obstruction, since 20% of calculi are radiolucent and are, therefore, undetectable on routine radiographs. Acute salivary gland infection can also be the cause of facial pain, but diagnosis is usually straightforward due to accompanying clinical signs which are typical of this condition.

Whenever pain is thought to be of salivary gland origin it must be fully investigated, since symptoms at these sites may indicate the presence of neoplasms, sometimes surprisingly small lesions.

Pain of vascular origin
Giant cell arteritis

Although rare, the vascular condition of most relevance to dental practitioners is giant cell arteritis, which is also known as temporal arteritis. The term 'temporal arteritis', however, is a poor one, since the condition can affect any head or neck artery and its occurrence is not restricted to temporal vessels. Patients with giant cell arteritis are usually elderly, have a degree of systemic upset and complain of jaw claudication. Jaw claudication is characterised by a cramp-like pain around the masseter, which occurs when the patient starts to eat. This pain prevents further jaw movement, which in turn leads to resolution of symptoms, allowing the patient to chew once again, for a limited period of time. Clinically, one or more extracranial vessels may be tender to palpation. The erythrocyte sedimentation rate (ESR) is usually greatly elevated and this finding, in combination with other clinical features, is sufficient for diagnosis. There is little merit in temporal artery biopsy, since the characteristic histological features are only present sporadically ('skip' lesions) and therefore multiple biopsies would be required to confirm diagnosis.

Giant cell arteritis should be regarded as an emergency, particularly when visual loss has occurred, since blindness of one eye can be followed by blindness of the other eye within 48 hours if high dose steroid therapy (prednisolone, 60–80 mg daily in divided doses) is not instituted. The usual contra-indications to the use of high dose steroid therapy should be observed and the patient should be given a steroid warning card, giving details of treatment prescribed. Giant cell arteritis is not necessarily a lifelong problem and therapy can gradually be reduced with time, provided the ESR falls and is sustained at a level normal for the age and sex of the patient.

Periodic migrainous neuralgia

Whilst it has not been established that periodic migrainous neuralgia is truly vascular in origin, it is useful to consider it under this heading. In this condition, patients usually complain of a severe pain around the eye, temple or malar region, which lasts from 30 to 120 minutes. The pain is episodic and the patient can go for days or weeks without attacks. During an attack the face on the affected side is flushed and there may be lacrimation or rhinorrhoea. Periodic migrainous neuralgia is one of the few non-dental pains which will wake a patient from their sleep. A useful indicator of the likely presence of this condition is the fact that patients report that alcohol, even in small amounts, can precipitate an attack. Treatment of choice is prophylactic indomethacin (75 mg nocte), although the use of ergotamine derivatives may also be successful.

Paroxysmal facial hemicrania

Paroxysmal facial hemicrania can present with symptoms identical to those of periodic migrainous neuralgia, although facial flushing and running of the eyes or nose is absent. This condition also responds well to indomethacin or ergotamine derivatives.

Pain of bony origin

Apart from trauma, there are a limited number of possible causes of pain of bony origin. Osteomata, including mandibular or palatal tori (fig. 4), can be traumatised and produce a complaint of localised, dull pain. The pain itself is self-limiting and is usually precipitated by hard foodstuffs or toothbrushing trauma.

Infection of bone is uncommon, except for the localised osteitis associated with a dry socket. Suppurative infections are also uncommon, but can be a complication of osteoradionecrosis. Although osteoradionecrosis is rarely seen nowadays, occasional cases do still occur, sometimes many years after irradiation (fig. 5).

Pain may be a feature of either primary or secondary tumours within bone. The nature of the pain varies, but has often been described as a constant dull ache, with no precipitating or relieving factors. The occurrence of a tumour is an important differential diagnosis of atypical facial pain, which may present with similar symptoms. Dental radiographs will usually detect the presence of a tumour within the maxilla or mandible (fig. 6). However, computerised tomography (fig. 7) or magnetic resonance imaging can also be invaluable in detecting tumour deposits, although the use of such high technology should not surpass information gained from clinical observation.

Patients suffering from Paget's disease may experience orofacial pain, owing to compression of branches of the trigeminal nerve as a result of bone formation at foramina of the base of the skull. Bone activity will also produce clinically obvious features such as enlargement of the skull (fig. 8) or widening and flattening of the hard palate. The presence of

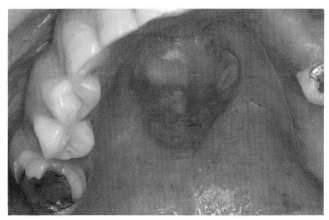

Fig. 4 Palatal tori with traumatised overlying mucosa.

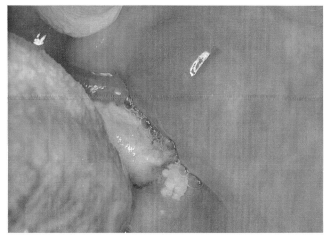

Fig. 5 Osteoradionecrosis present as an area of ulceration in the third molar region.

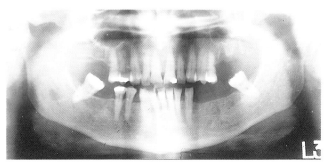

Fig. 6 Radiolucency in right ramus of mandible due to metastatic spread of a breast tumour.

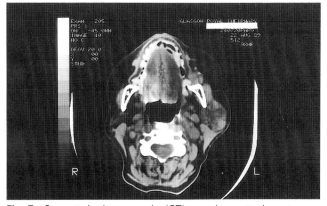

Fig. 7 Computerised tomography (CT) scan demonstrating a tumour in the left parotid gland.

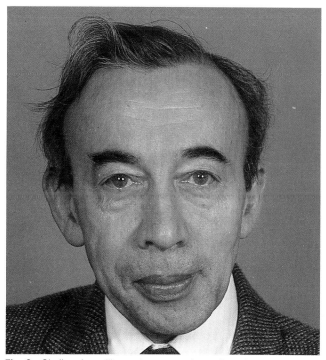

Fig. 8 Skull and maxillary enlargement due to Paget's disease.

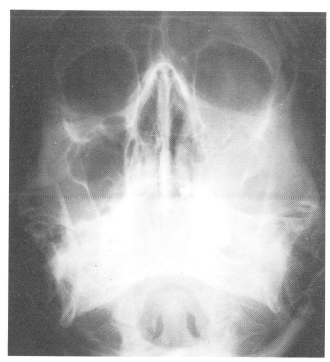

Fig. 9 Radiopacity of the left maxillary antrum due to the presence of a neoplasm.

Paget's disease can be confirmed by haematological detection of a raised alkaline phosphatase level of bony origin. Radiographs may reveal the presence of a 'cotton wool' appearance to the calvarium and hypercementosis around the roots of teeth.

Pain from the maxillary sinus

The intimate relationship between the maxillary air sinus and the upper posterior dentition can cause problems when trying to differentiate between pain of sinus origin and that of dental origin. Radiographs (fig. 9) or computerised tomographs of the sinuses and teeth can be of assistance, but, as always, a good history is essential. Symptoms which would support the presence of sinusitis include toothache-like pain affecting several upper posterior teeth, absence of tenderness to percussion of the teeth, and increased severity of symptoms during movements of the head, particularly on bending forward. In the short term, antibiotic therapy, such as amoxycillin or tetracycline, will resolve the infection and consequently relieve the symptoms of maxillary sinusitis. If the patient suffers from recurrent episodes, then referral for a surgical opinion should be considered.

The frontal, ethmoidal or sphenoidal air sinuses can all also have pathology associated with them. Branches of the trigeminal nerve innervate the lining of these sinuses, in addition to supplying sensation of the skin of the face. There is therefore considerable potential for referred pain to cause orofacial symptoms.

Pain from the temporomandibular joint

There has probably been more written about temporomandibular joint dysfunction syndrome than almost any other painful condition which may present to the dental practitioner. A variety of terms including Costen's syndrome, myofascial pain dysfunction syndrome and facial arthromyalgia, have been used to describe the situation where pain arises from the temporomandibular joint apparatus.

Simplistically, it is useful to differentiate TMJ disease from TMJ dysfunction at the outset. In cases of TMJ disease, there is an anatomical abnormality of the joint which should be detectable on radiographs, tomography or arthrography. An example of such an abnormality is the presence of osteophytes arising from the condylar head, which give rise to pain on mandibular movement. Although conservative treatment with analgesics can help in this situation, surgical intervention is usually required in the long term.

In contrast to TMJ disease, radiographs fail to reveal any abnormality in TMJ dysfunction, since it is a functional disorder. It could be argued that radiographic investigation is not required when clinical signs and symptoms are sufficiently supportive of TMJ dysfunction. Characteristic features of the condition are trismus, pain over the condylar region and tenderness of the muscles of mastication. Parafunctional habits such as clenching or grinding appear to be important in TMJ dysfunction and, therefore, patients often wake with the pain in the morning or report that symptoms develop as the day goes on. It has been claimed that stress or anxiety trigger parafunctional habits and, interestingly, TMJ dysfunction appears to be more frequent in younger people, especially at times of examination or other stressful life events.

When active treatment is required, our preferred management of TMJ dysfunction is the provision of a hard acrylic splint which opens the bite by approximately 2 mm. Adam's cribs should be incorporated to provide retention, and the appliance should cover all the occlusal surfaces of the standing teeth (fig. 10). When fitted, the splint should achieve even occlusal contact in centric relation and during lateral excursion. Clearly, TMJ dysfunction is not a lifelong condition, although patients usually need to wear the splint (at night only) for several months. Some clinicians prefer the use of soft vacuum formed splints, but these are bulky and cannot easily be modified to achieve even occlusal contact.

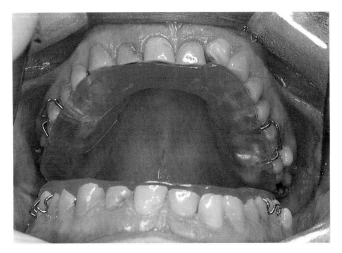

Fig. 10 Acrylic splint used for the treatment of patients with TMJ dysfunction or migraine on waking.

Selective occlusal grinding of the teeth for the treatment of TMJ dysfunction has its advocates, although this approach is by no means universally accepted. However, the presence of obvious occlusal interference, particularly in recently placed restorations, should be eliminated.

Finally, acrylic splint therapy can also be of benefit in the treatment of migraine, although it is important to establish that patients truly have migraine and therefore suffer from severe prolonged headaches (6–36 hours) with associated nausea, vomiting or photophobia. The patients with migraine who appear to benefit most from splint therapy are those who suffer from attacks on or within 1–2 hours of waking.

Pain of central nervous system origin
Trigeminal neuralgia

Trigeminal neuralgia is commoner in women than in men and can affect any division of the trigeminal nerve. Interestingly, the maxillary or mandibular division, particularly on the right side, appears to be most frequently involved. Classically, trigger factors such as smiling, eating or touching the skin, have been described in this condition, although in practice these are present in the minority of patients. The pain is described as 'lancinating' or 'electric-shock like', and is of such severity that even the most stoical of patients will describe attacks as '10 out of 10', 'the worst pain I have ever experienced', which 'stops them in their tracks'. Prior to the onset of the characteristic symptoms of trigeminal neuralgia, approximately 20% of patients have an entirely different pain, known as pretrigeminal neuralgia, which affects the teeth and can be confused with pulpitis, cracked tooth syndrome or dentine hypersensitivity.

Both trigeminal and pretrigeminal neuralgia respond well to carbamazepine therapy if used properly. Since carbamazepine is not an analgesic but a membrane stabilising drug, it is crucial that patients recognise the importance of adhering to the prescribed regime. An initial dose of 100 mg t.i.d. should be prescribed and this may be increased in 100 mg increments every 3–4 days until the pain is controlled. Patients usually become asymptomatic on a total daily dose of 400–800 mg. It is prudent to take a blood sample (10 mg clotted) prior to placing any patient on carbamazepine therapy, in order to assess liver enzymes, since hepatotoxicity, although rare, can occur. There is little point in monitoring

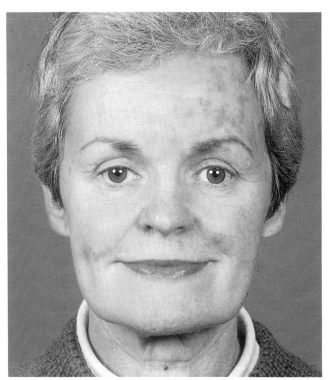

Fig. 11 Post-herpetic pigmentation affecting the skin supplied by the left ophthalmic division of the trigeminal nerve.

blood levels of the drug during treatment, unless overdose is suspected, since the laboratory reference range only applies to the use of carbamazepine in the management of epilepsy. In addition, the laboratory will not routinely measure the active metabolites of the drug, in particular epoxides.

The main reason for failure of carbamazepine therapy is poor patient compliance with the prescribed dose schedules. Phenytoin may also be used in the management of trigeminal neuralgia and it should be considered for those patients in whom carbamazepine is ineffective. Cryotherapy and a variety of surgical options, including intracranial procedures, are also available, but these should be reserved for occasions when drug therapy has not been successful.

Rare causes of orofacial pain of central nervous system origin include acoustic neuromas, intracranial neoplasms and multiple sclerosis, all of which can, on occasions, present as trigeminal neuralgia.

Glossopharyngeal neuralgia

The nature and symptoms of glossopharyngeal neuralgia are very similar to those of trigeminal neuralgia. However, in this condition the distribution of the ninth cranial nerve is affected and, therefore, patients complain of a unilateral pain involving the posterior third of the tongue, and the tonsillar region or the ear. Management of glossopharyngeal neuralgia should be based on the use of carbamazepine.

Pain of infective origin
Post-herpetic neuralgia

Reactivation of *Varicella zoster* virus is responsible for the condition known as shingles (herpes zoster). Following an episode of shingles, a patient may suffer from either residual pigmentation (fig. 11) or post-herpetic neuralgia. The post-inflammatory pigmented lesions are limited to the skin supplied by affected branches of the trigeminal nerve and may

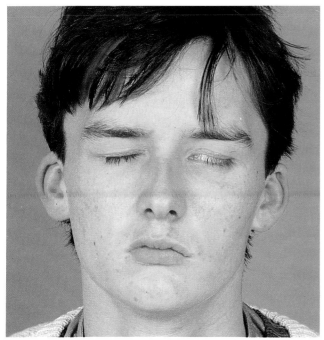

Fig. 12 Left-sided facial nerve palsy in a teenager with Ramsay-Hunt syndrome.

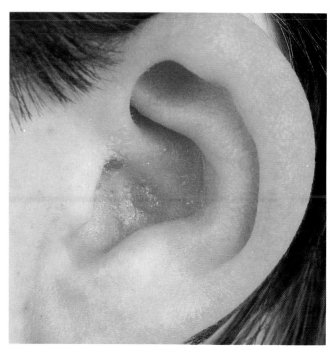

Fig. 13 Vesicular lesions in the external auditory meatus of the patient seen in figure 12.

produce an aesthetic problem for some time. The pain due to post-herpetic neuralgia is intense and may be associated with symptoms of hyperaesthesia and paraesthesia. The condition tends to affect older patients and can be particularly distressing, since it may be totally resistant to a range of drug treatments, including tricyclic antidepressants. It would be a considerable advance if acyclovir, an antiviral agent used to treat herpes zoster, could also be proven to minimise the development of post-herpetic neuralgia.

Ramsay-Hunt syndrome

Ramsay-Hunt syndrome is characterised by a combination of clinical signs and symptoms which are due to *Varicella zoster* infection of the geniculate ganglion. Patients generally complain of pain, vesicular cutaneous eruptions in the outer ear and facial nerve palsy (figs 12 and 13). There are differing opinions on the best treatment of Ramsay-Hunt syndrome. Although some authorities believe no successful treatment is available, it would seem appropriate to provide antiviral therapy, in the form of acyclovir, to limit viral activity. In addition, it has been suggested that the use of corticosteroid therapy will reduce the inflammatory oedema which is probably responsible for the facial nerve palsy. Active and rapid treatment of facial nerve palsy is important, since, if untreated, the defect may be permanent and can present a very distressing cosmetic problem for the patient.

Pain of psychogenic origin

Orofacial pain is a component of a variety of psychiatric disorders, ranging from hypochondriacal individuals who use orofacial pain as gain, to anxious individuals who somatise their complaints in terms of organic disease.

Atypical facial pain

Unfortunately, the term atypical facial pain is often misused and is applied to painful conditions which either do not fit into any other disease category or cross anatomical boundaries. This is unfortunate since the original descriptions of atypical facial pain were quite specific, consisting of a constant pain (nothing makes it better, nothing makes it worse) which is usually localised over the maxilla and frequently affects middle-aged women. In addition, the patients will usually complain of headache, backache, dysfunctional uterine bleeding, irritable bowel syndrome and itchy skin. Depression and anxiety are likely to be major factors in atypical facial pain, but without experience in these areas it is difficult to detect the presence of these components by clinical interview alone. The Hospital Anxiety and Depression (HAD) scale (see chapter 3) is a useful tool in confirming the presence of either anxiety or depression and may reveal surprisingly high scores for these factors in apparently normal individuals. A major advantage of the HAD scale is that its use does not require any specialist training. Tricyclic antidepressants are very effective in controlling atypical facial pain, and dothiepin (75 mg nocte) is the drug of choice. It is a matter of some controversy as to whether it is the antidepressant action of the tricyclic drug which controls the pain or whether relief is achieved due to some other mechanism.

Clearly, organic disease, particularly the presence of an antral tumour (fig. 9), should be excluded when the patient complains of a constant pain over the maxillary sinus.

Miscellaneous conditions

It is not possible, in a brief description of orofacial pain, to be comprehensive and include rare conditions such as Eagle's syndrome and neck–tongue syndrome. Fortunately, however, owing to their rarity, it is extremely unlikely that these syndromes will be encountered in general dental practice.

6
Orofacial allergic reactions

Allergic reactions may produce a variety of clinical signs and symptoms. It is now apparent that the occurrence of lip swelling, oral ulceration or mucosal white patches may be due to a sensitivity to components of dental materials, drugs, toothpastes or constituents of food and drink. Although such problems do not occur frequently, it is important to identify any factor which may be responsible for orofacial lesions, since elimination of the allergen will usually lead to rapid resolution of symptoms.

In recent years there has been an increasing amount of interest concerning allergy, and a number of agents have been proposed as being involved in allergic phenomena. However, it is essential that scientific research is undertaken prior to implicating any particular substance as a significant allergen. It is therefore our policy to confirm suspected allergies by the use of cutaneous patch testing and immunological investigations. It is also important that the patch testing is undertaken by a dermatologist who is experienced both in the technique and interpretation of results.

Clearly, allergy investigation is not a first line of approach for patients with orofacial complaints. There are, however, certain diseases, particularly orofacial granulomatosis and lichenoid eruptions, which would support the early institution of allergy tests.

Background to patch testing
Patch testing is based on use of the Standard European Series of environmental allergens such as metals, rubbers, cosmetics and foodstuffs. Additional substances may also be included as part of the test, depending on the patient's signs, symptoms and history. In brief, there are two types of test, both of which consist of applying substances to areas of normal skin on the patient's back using aluminium discs held in place by hypo-allergenic tape (fig. 1). One set of test sites are observed for up to 6 hours after application, to see if there is an immediate Type I response (urticaria). A duplicate set of tests are examined after 2 and 4 days, to detect a Type IV reaction (allergic).

If a food-related allergen is identified, then a trained dietician can provide the patient with a diet which excludes the suspected allergen. If the allergen is not a foodstuff but an environmental agent, such as nickel, then the patient is given appropriate advice on avoidance by a Nursing Liaison Sister. It is sometimes necessary to visit the patient's home or place of work to ensure that all allergens can be avoided.

Following counselling, the patient should be reviewed regularly, at approximately 3-monthly intervals, to monitor their progress and give further support as necessary.

Orofacial granulomatosis
Orofacial granulomatosis (OFG) has previously been described as oral Crohn's disease or, when accompanied by facial nerve palsy and fissured tongue, the Melkersson-Rosenthal syndrome. For reasons which are not clear at the present time, OFG is relatively common in the West of Scotland, and in the past 10 years more than 150 patients with the condition have been referred to the Oral Medicine Clinic in Glasgow. There appears to be an equal distribution between males and females, with symptoms usually appearing in either the second or third decade.

In the absence of any definite history of weight loss or bowel symptoms, we do not feel that patients should be subjected to full gastrointestinal screening for Crohn's disease, since investigations, such as barium meal with follow-through, sigmoidoscopy and rectal biopsy can be distressing, particularly to children. In our experience, patients who present with OFG rarely progress to develop the gastrointestinal features of Crohn's disease.

The cardinal clinical features of OFG are facial or lip swelling (fig. 2), angular cheilitis (fig. 3), a full width gingivitis (fig. 4), oral ulceration (fig. 5), mucosal tags (fig. 6) and a

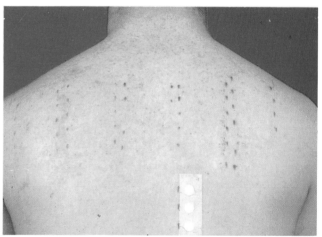

Fig. 1 Appearance of a patient's back during patch testing. Some test strips have been removed, but coded marking indicates the exact site of exposure.

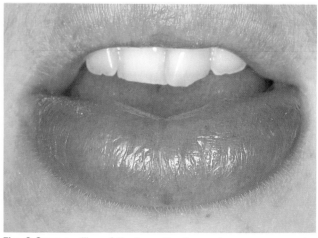

Fig. 2 Gross swelling of the lower lip, the most common presenting symptom of OFG.

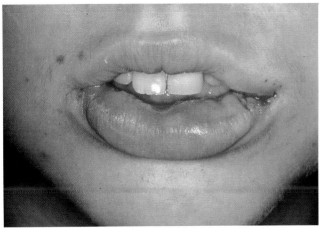

Fig. 3 Angular cheilitis, which occurs in approximately 20% of patients with OFG.

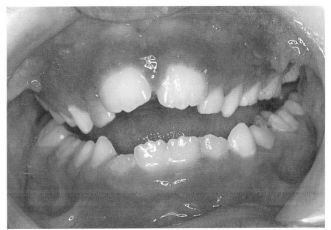

Fig. 4 Full-width gingivitis characteristic of OFG.

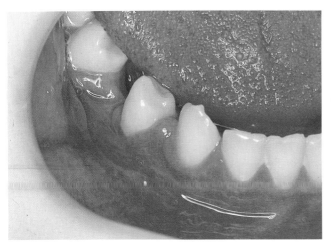

Fig. 5 Oral ulceration in a patient with OFG.

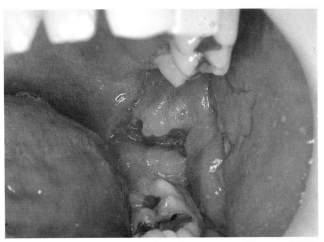

Fig. 6 Mucosal tags in the retromolar region are a typical feature of OFG.

cobblestoned oral mucosa (fig. 7). Not all these features are clinically obvious in every patient, and there may be wide individual variations in signs and symptoms. Facial or lip swelling is the most common presenting complaint.

Intra-oral biopsy down to muscle characteristically reveals non-caseating granulomata and lymphoedema. Indeed, it is lymphoedema which is responsible for the dramatic lip or facial swelling seen in some patients. Although all clinically involved sites are likely to show these histological features,

the buccal mucosa is the preferred area for biopsy, since this site is easily accessible and causes the patient minimum discomfort. Biopsy of an already oedematous lip is likely to cause the patient further distress, owing to the likelihood of post-operative swelling.

Once a clinical diagnosis of OFG has been made, then the patient should be referred for patch testing. In addition to the Standard European Series, elements such as cinnamonaldehyde, benzoic acid, other benzoates and chocolate should be included when OFG is suspected.

Prior to patch testing, it is often useful to question the patient on known allergies or previous history of eczema, asthma or hayfever, since there appears to be an association between OFG and atopy. In addition, aspects of dietary habits, in particular frequent intake of cinnamon and benzoates, may be clues since experience has shown that these elements are often involved in OFG. Cinnamon is a frequent flavouring agent and benzoic acid is used as a food preservative. Inclusion of cinnamon or benzoate in foodstuffs is usually indicated on labelling; benzoates are designated by the E numbers, E210–E219. It is helpful to instruct patients suspected of having OFG to avoid these substances during the period whilst waiting for patch tesing, since it may lead to some reduction in symptoms. Systemic terfenadine at a dosage of 60 mg once or twice daily can also be helpful in reducing symptoms without producing the side-effect of drowsiness associated with other antihistamines. Once an allergen has been detected, the patient should be given appropriate exclusion advice and followed up at regular (3-monthly) intervals. Resolution of symptoms should occur within 6–18 months (fig. 8).

Burning mouth syndrome

As mentioned in the third chapter of this book, some patients, particularly those with Type 3 burning mouth syndrome, may have an allergic component to their complaint. Characteristically, such individuals have wide variations in the pattern of the complaint, with asymptomatic periods accompanied by times of severe burning affecting unusual sites such as floor of mouth and throat. Allergens which have been identified in patients with burning mouth syndrome include propylene glycol, sorbic acid, benzoates and cinnamonaldehyde. However, exclusion of these substances does not always result

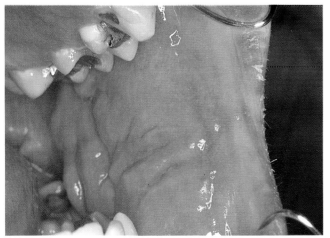

Fig. 7 Cobblestone appearance of the buccal mucosa in a patient with OFG.

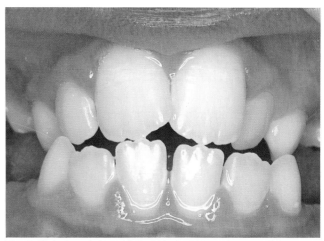

Fig. 8 Clinical resolution of full width gingivitis in the case of the patient shown in figure 4 following institution of a benzoic acid-free diet.

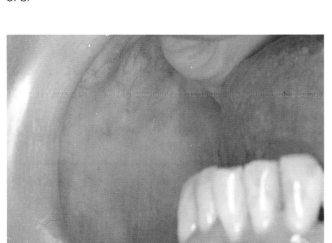

Fig. 9 Right buccal mucosa of a patient suffering from a lichenoid reaction.

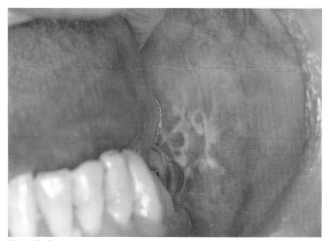

Fig. 10 Striated white patch affecting buccal mucosa of the patient shown in figure 9. Note asymmetrical distribution of the condition.

in total resolution of symptoms. In addition, there are occasions when no allergen is found. In these circumstances, emotional instability is likely to be a factor and this should be managed along with the other known aetiological factors of burning mouth syndrome.

Lichenoid reaction
Intra-oral lichenoid reactions may be due either to systemic drug therapy or a local reaction to the mercury component of amalgam restorations. Although the list of drugs implicated in lichenoid reactions is long and ever-increasing, the most commonly involved agents are antihypertensives, gold, hypoglycaemics and non-steroidal anti-inflammatory drugs. Lichenoid reactions do not have a pathognomic clinical appearance and can mimic lichen planus. Lack of symmetry (figs 9 and 10), involvement of the palate (fig. 11) or a history of recent or continuing drug therapy, are, however, suggestive of a lichenoid reaction rather than lichen planus.

Mucosal biopsy is helpful, since an experienced oral pathologist may be able to detect features which are suggestive of a lichenoid reaction rather than those seen in lichen planus. In addition, a haematological specimen (10 ml clotted sample) in a plain tube can be sent for indirect immunofluorescence examination; a positive 'string of pearls' effect would support a lichenoid eruption. However, even

with information from these investigations, it can sometimes be difficult to prove that a drug has caused a lichenoid reaction. In practice it is often not possible to stop a systemic drug, such as an antihypertensive, and observe resolution of symptoms. If the oral lesions are causing concern or discomfort, the option of using a structurally unrelated drug with similar therapeutic effects should be considered, following direct liaison with the patient's medical practitioner. If the suspected drug was responsible and this course of action is followed, then resolution of symptoms should occur within 2 to 3 months (fig. 12).

It was suggested in one recent study that as many as one in three patients who were originally thought to have erosive lichen planus actually had a patch test confirmed lichenoid reaction to amalgam. The occurrence of lichenoid reactions due to amalgam restorations may not, therefore, be as uncommon as originally thought. Clinically, reactions to amalgam usually affect the buccal mucosa or tongue in areas which are closely associated with older corroded amalgam restorations (fig. 13). Patch testing should demonstrate sensitivity to amalgam and specifically ammoniated mercury, which is the usual allergen. Replacement of amalgam restorations with composite materials is likely to produce clinical resolution within a few weeks (fig. 14). It is obviously advisable to confirm such sensitivity by the use of patch

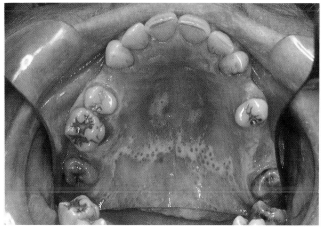

Fig. 11 Lichenoid reaction which developed in the palate of a patient, following institution of methyldopa therapy.

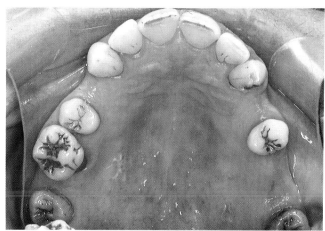

Fig. 12 Considerable clinical improvement of the lichenoid reaction shown in figure 11, following discontinuation of methyldopa therapy.

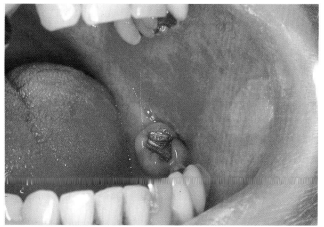

Fig. 13 Lichenoid reaction affecting buccal mucosa adjacent to a large amalgam restoration.

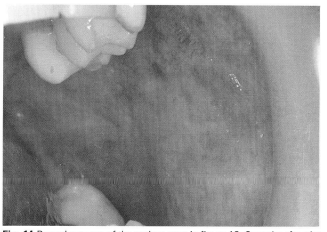

Fig. 14 Buccal mucosa of the patient seen in figure 13, 2 weeks after the replacement of amalgam restoration with a composite material.

testing prior to subjecting any patient to the replacement of large or numerous amalgam restorations.

At the present time there is no compelling evidence for a link between amalgam restorations and systemic disease such as myalgic encephalitis (post-viral syndrome) or multiple sclerosis. It is understandable, however, that patients with these conditions attend the dental surgery if they read or hear about such associations in the general media.

Denture materials

Adverse reactions to denture materials, such as acrylic or cobalt chromium, are rare. In our experience, such suspected reactions are almost invariably accompanied by other changes in the oral mucosa.

Patients with acrylic dentures who have an allergy to methylmethacrylate confirmed by patch testing will benefit from the provision of replacement appliances constructed of polycarbonate or nylon. Patients with cobalt chrome dentures may be found to be sensitive to nickel. In these circumstances, nickel-free cobalt chromium is available for the construction of alternative appliances.

Erythema multiforme

Erythema multiforme presents with the acute development of widespread oral ulceration (fig. 15), blood-crusted lips and

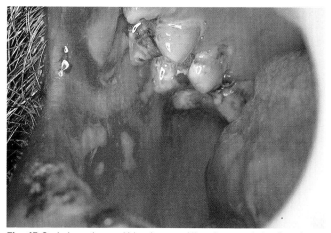

Fig. 15 Oral ulceration and blood-crusted lips characteristic of erythema multiforme.

perhaps skin lesions (fig. 16). Unless there are known precipitating factors such as drug therapy or infection, patients characteristically have two or three episodes of reducing severity over a period of 2 to 3 years. However, cases of sensitivity to food preservatives would appear to be an important precipitating factor in cases of recurrent erythema multiforme where severity of symptoms remains constant.

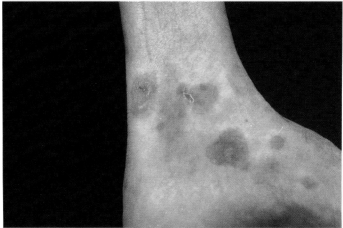

Fig. 16 Cutaneous lesions of erythema multiforme affecting the foot.

Local anaesthetics

It is not uncommon for patients to suspect that they have an allergy to local anaesthetics. The scenario is usually of an adverse reaction such as nausea or a feeling of lightheadedness during or immediately following dental treatment. In the absence of changes, such as skin rash, true allergy is unlikely. It is far more common for symptoms to be due to either inadvertent intravenous introduction of anaesthetic which produces a transient tachycardia, or patient anxiety which precipitates an episode of syncope. Whenever allergy to local anaesthetic is suspected, direct challenge should be performed rather than patch testing, since the reaction involved is a Type I hypersensitivity and not a delayed Type IV reaction. It is essential that such a challenge is undertaken in a hospital setting, where resuscitation facilities are immediately available, since if true allergy is present the patient may experience anaphylactic shock. Hopefully, in the future, a radioallergosorbent (RAST) test for serum IgE levels towards the group of local anaesthetics may be available. This would obviously be useful, since it only involves the taking of a blood sample and would, therefore, avoid the dangers associated with direct challenge.

Angioedema

This uncommon condition is either inherited as a C-1 esterase inhibitor deficiency or can be secondary to drug therapy, particularly antihypertensive agents. Patients will report the sudden onset and presence of areas of facial or tongue swelling. Tongue swelling can be dramatic and endanger the airway. Specialist investigations are required on these patients and they are also probably best treated in a hospital setting, since minor trauma may precipitate attacks.

7

White patches

Certain conditions of the oral mucosa may present as white patches. Although the majority of white patches are benign, some lesions are associated with premalignancy or malignancy. Unfortunately, the presence of any sinister lesion cannot be assessed by clinical appearance alone and accurate diagnosis (involving biopsy) is therefore mandatory whenever there is uncertainty about the clinical diagnosis of an oral white patch.

White sponge naevus

White sponge naevus is a developmental condition which affects males and females equally since it is inherited in an autosomal dominant manner. The developmental nature of white sponge naevus would seem to suggest that it could be detected in early life, but, surprisingly, it is not unusual for affected individuals to be first diagnosed in adolescence. Questioning will often reveal that other members of the family have similar oral lesions. The extent of clinical signs is variable, but large areas of the floor of the mouth and buccal sulcus are often involved (fig. 1). In addition, areas of nasal or vaginal mucosa may be affected. A mucosal biopsy should be undertaken to confirm the clinical diagnosis and to exclude the presence of the rare but serious developmental condition, dyskeratosis congenita, in which malignant transformation has been reported. Once diagnosed histologically, patients with white sponge naevus should be reassured about the benign nature of the condition.

Traumatic lesions

Traumatic injury of the oral mucosa due to chemical or thermal irritation can produce a variety of characteristic clinical white patches. In children a cheek biting habit may have a similar clinical appearance to white sponge naevus, although differentiation between the two conditions is relatively easy since cheek biting will be restricted to areas which can be physically chewed (fig. 2). Placement of an aspirin adjacent to a painful tooth will initially produce a white patch, but this sloughs off in 1–2 days, leaving an irregular erosion which heals normally. Chronic irritation can produce a white appearance of any area of the mucosa, although the palate is often affected in relation to a chronic pipe-smoking habit; this is known as nicotinic stomatitis or smoker's keratosis (fig. 3). It is generally accepted that tobacco usage is associated with an increased risk of oral malignancy. Patients with nicotinic stomatitis should be actively discouraged from smoking, since discontinuation of the habit should result in resolution of their white patches. Sometimes an area of ulceration due to a thermal burn may develop within a pre-existing nicotinic stomatitis (fig. 4) and it is obviously important, in these circumstances, to ensure that the lesion resolves within 2 weeks. Although the palate is a rare site for malignant change, it is essential to exclude the presence of a carcinoma if the lesion persists beyond this time.

As mentioned previously, chronic physical irritation is characterised by hyperkeratosis of the mucosa, limited to the areas being traumatised, with a sharp demarcation from the surrounding normal tissues (fig. 5). It is always good clinical

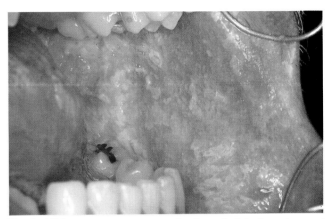
Fig. 1 White sponge naevus extending buccally into the sulcus and posteriorly into the retromolar region.

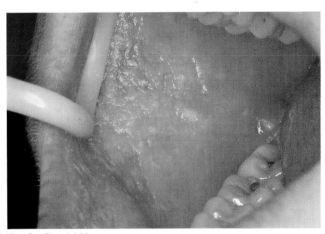
Fig. 2 Cheek biting.

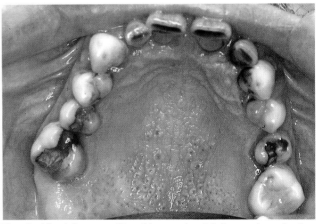
Fig. 3 Nicotinic stomatitis with associated inflammation of minor salivary gland ducts.

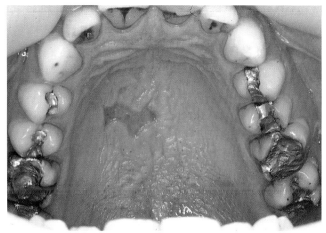

Fig. 4 Thermal burn arising in the palate of a patient with a pre-existing nicotinic stomatitis.

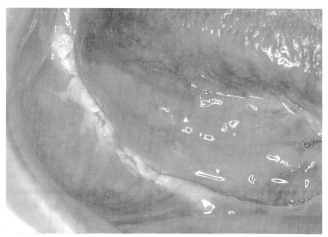

Fig. 5 Well demarcated white patch on the crest of the lower alveolar ridge in a patient who did not wear a lower full denture.

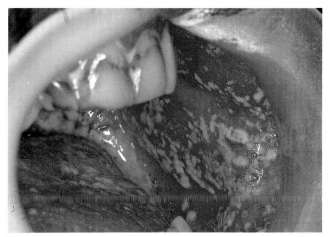

Fig. 6 Acute pseudomembranous candidosis in a patient receiving broad spectrum antibiotic therapy.

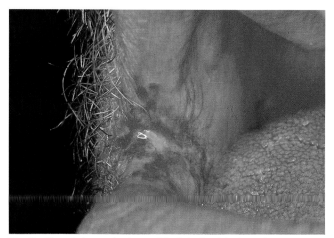

Fig. 7 Chronic hyperplastic candidosis in the right buccal commissure.

practice to eliminate the traumatic cause, such as an over-extended denture or rough tooth surface, and to ensure that the appearance of the mucosa returns entirely to normal within 2–3 weeks. Any white patch suspected of being caused by trauma and persisting after this time must be biopsied.

Candidal infection

The two candidoses of importance in the context of oral white patches are pseudomembranous candidosis (thrush) and chronic hyperplastic candidosis (candidal leukoplakia or *Candida*-associated leukoplakia).

Pseudomembranous candidosis is characterised, as its name suggests, by extensive white pseudomembranes consisting of desquamated epithelial cells, fungal hyphae and fibrin (fig. 6). This membrane can be scraped off with a spatula or swab to expose an underlying erythematous mucosa. Diagnosis is usually straightforward, although it should be confirmed microbiologically, either by staining of a smear from the affected area or by culture of a swab or an oral rinse. Whenever pseudomembranous candidosis, or indeed any form of oral candidosis, is diagnosed it is necessary to consider why candidal infection has arisen. In some patients, broad spectrum antibiotic therapy or steroid therapy, in particular the use of inhalers, can precipitate candidal proliferation, whilst in others it is a result of an immunological abnormality (ranging from neutropenia to HIV infection). In addition, haematological deficiencies,

blood dyscrasias or undiagnosed diabetes mellitus have been implicated in predisposing to oral candidosis. Therefore, full investigation is warranted in all patients and referral for appropriate counselling is essential if HIV infection is suspected.

Treatment of pseudomembranous candidosis involves eliminating any predisposing factors and the institution of antifungal therapy, such as nystatin pastilles or amphotericin lozenges (dissolved in the mouth four times a day) for a period of up to 2 weeks after clinical resolution. Nystatin suspension can be used when pseudomembranous candidosis occurs in neonates. Recently, systemic triazole therapy (fluconazole, 50 mg tablet daily for 7 days) has been found to be effective in eradicating intra-oral candidosis in immunocompromised patients.

Chronic hyperplastic candidosis characteristically occurs bilaterally in the commissure region (fig. 7) as homogeneous or speckled lesions. As previously mentioned, the presence of any underlying systemic disease should be excluded when candidosis is suspected, but in chronic hyperplastic lesions smoking also appears to be an important local factor. Traditionally, the condition has been treated by antifungal therapy given topically for periods of up to 3 months. Unfortunately, compliance with this prolonged drug regime is likely to be poor and eradication of *Candida* is therefore unlikely to occur. It would also appear that clinical resolution depends on whether the patient stops smoking. Poor compliance may well partly explain the known incidence of malignant change associated with hyperplastic candidosis. In view of this, it may be more appropriate to prescribe systemic fluconazole (50 mg daily for 7 days), since it has been shown that this approach is effective in the treatment of chronic hyperplastic candidosis (fig. 8). It is important, however, to maintain any patient treated in this way on a long-term follow-up to determine whether the risk of malignant change (presently of the order of 7% in a 10-year period) is reduced.

Bacterial infection

Leukoplakia of the dorsal surface of the tongue is a recognised clinical feature of tertiary syphilis. In the past this condition was strongly associated with the development of oral cancer in the mid-line of the tongue. However, detection and effective treatment of syphilis at early stages now means that syphilitic leukoplakia is extremely rare.

Viral infection

The most important lesion which has been associated with viral infection is hairy leukoplakia. This condition is discussed in detail elsewhere in this book, but is included here since it characteristically presents as white patches on the lateral border of the tongue. Since hairy leukoplakia is almost exclusively associated with HIV infection, biopsy of white patches on the lateral border of the tongue is mandatory.

Neoplastic and premalignant lesions

Oral malignancy and premalignancy still represent a great clinical challenge, since mortality from oral cancer is largely unchanged this century. Mortality is still over 50% after 5 years and it appears that oral cancer is increasing in prevalence.

Studies which have tried to establish the aetiological factors which are involved in the development of oral cancer have used the clinical term 'leukoplakia'. By definition leukoplakia should be used to describe 'a white patch' or plaque that cannot be characterised, clinically or pathologically, as any other disease. Leukoplakia is a clinical term only and has no histological connotations since very often the 'any other disease' can be established following biopsy. However, widespread clinical use of the term leukoplakia has resulted in an association with the presence of epithelial dysplasia and premalignant potential. It has become apparent that the most significant aetiological factors in leukoplakia and subsequently oral cancer are tobacco usage, alcohol ingestion, nutritional deficiency and candidal infection.

The clinical presentation of leukoplakia can vary from minimal localised lesions (fig. 9) to extensive involvement of the mucosa (fig. 10). It is important to appreciate that the degree of dysplasia or presence of carcinomatous change bears little relationship to the clinical appearance. The presence of all potential aetiological factors must be taken into account in the management of any patient with leukoplakia and therefore mucosal biopsy, haematological investigation and microbiological tests are mandatory. The biopsy should be performed primarily to exclude the presence of carcinoma. The biopsy material should therefore be taken from an area which looks clinically 'worst'. In this respect it is now generally accepted that erythematous and speckled areas are more worrying than uniform white plaques.

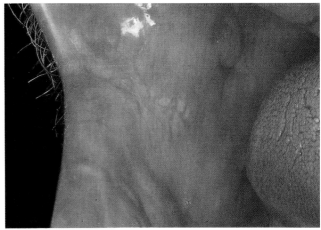

Fig. 8 Buccal mucosa of the patient shown in figure 7, 2 weeks after treatment with fluconazole.

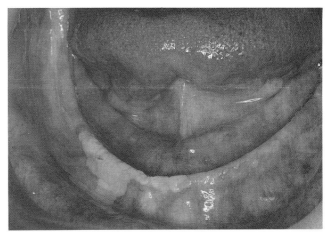

Fig. 9 Localised leukoplakia affecting the lower alveolar ridge.

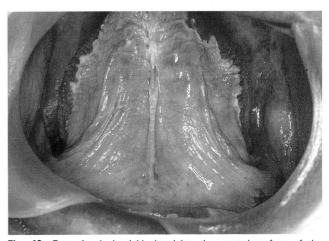

Fig. 10 Extensive leukoplakia involving the ventral surface of the tongue and floor of the mouth.

If carcinoma is not present, the specimen should be examined for evidence of dysplasia which, if present, can be graded as mild, moderate or severe. It is our policy to arrange immediate surgical removal of all lesions which are reported as showing evidence of severe dysplasia, whereas mildly or moderately dysplastic lesions can be treated more conservatively. However, the clinician cannot feel any 'safer' with a patient who has a mildly dysplastic lesion as opposed to moderate dysplasia, since the presence of any degree of dysplasia greatly increases the likelihood of malignant change. Management should include appropriate advice on

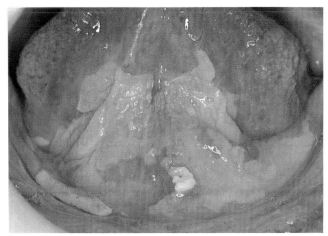

Fig. 11 Mildly dysplastic leukoplakia in the floor of the mouth and ventral surface of the tongue, prior to 10 days topical bleomycin therapy.

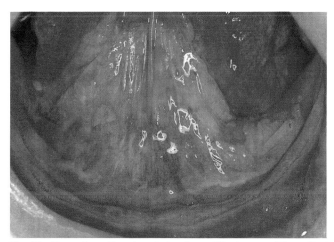

Fig. 12 Floor of mouth and ventral surface of the tongue of the patient shown in figure 11, 2 years later.

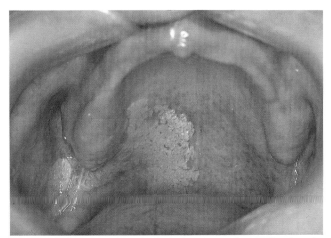

Fig. 13 Oral cancer arising in the soft palate and extending into the faucial region.

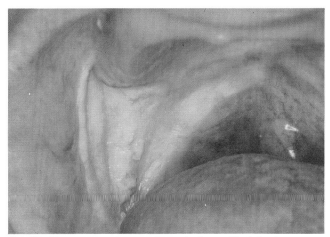

Fig. 14 The same patient as shown in figure 13, following tumour excision and repair using a skin graft.

elimination of smoking or drinking habits, investigation and correction of any haematological abnormality and eradication of candidal infection. Rebiopsy of the white patch after 3 months is essential in order to assess any histological progression or regression. Hopefully, if the previous aetiological factors have been corrected then improvement will have occurred. If this is the case then the patient should be kept under continued review (6-monthly). If a lesion is histologically unchanged after 3 months, then the options are either to keep the patient under 6-monthly review (although no more than 2 years should pass before rebiopsy) or to consider active treatment such as surgical removal, cryosurgery, laser therapy, or topical chemotherapy. It is probably wise to surgically remove small, easily accessible lesions. Topical bleomycin is our preferred treatment for extensive white patches or those which would be difficult to treat surgically. Bleomycin is an anti-cancer drug which can be dissolved in dimethylsulphoxide and applied topically at a dose of 15 mg a day for 10 consecutive days. Clinical response to this form of treatment is good and can give sustained effects over long-term follow-up (figs 11 and 12).

If a patient develops an oral cancer (fig. 13), then our policy is to arrange definitive surgical excision (fig. 14). However, opinions do differ and the use of radiotherapy or chemotherapy as adjuncts to surgery may also be considered, depending on individual cases. The development of one

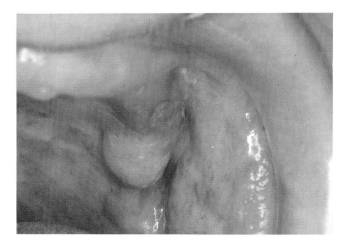

Fig. 15 The same patient as shown in figure 14, 2 years following initial surgery. A second primary carcinoma has arisen in the upper left molar region.

primary oral cancer confers a high risk of developing further primary lesions (fig. 15) and such patients therefore need careful long-term follow-up, involving thorough examination of the mucosa at regular 6-monthly intervals.

In the context of oral cancer, a patient may have an oral white patch as a result of the use of a skin graft to repair the site of tumour excision (fig. 16). In such circumstances the diagnosis of a white patch would be obvious from the patient's history.

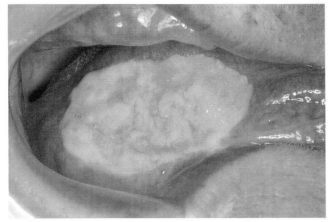

Fig. 16 Split thickness skin graft used to repair defects following excision of squamous cell carcinoma of the right lateral border of the tongue.

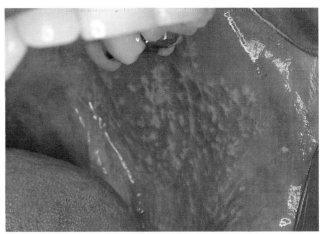

Fig. 17 Reticular lichen planus of the left buccal mucosa.

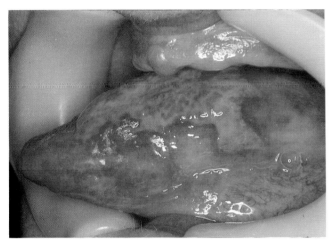

Fig. 18 Erosive lichen planus on the dorsal and lateral surfaces of the tongue.

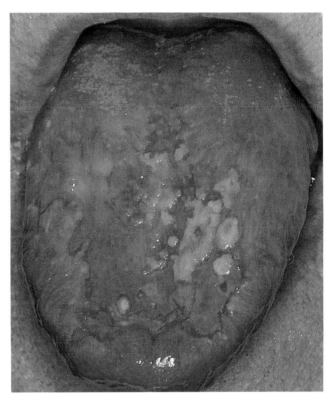

Fig. 20 Atrophic lichen planus.

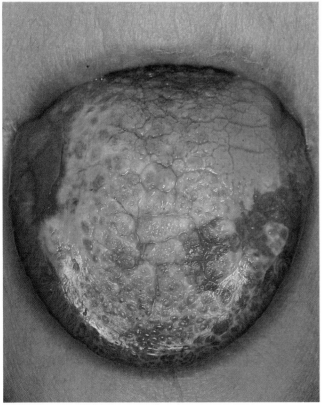

Fig. 19 Plaque-like lichen planus of the dorsal surface of the tongue.

Lichen planus

Lichen planus is a mucocutaneous disorder which affects the oral mucosa and/or skin of 1–2% of the population in the United Kingdom. Although, not surprisingly, there is an apparent predominance of oral lesions in patients attending dental surgeries or oral medicine clinics, skin lesions are seen just as frequently at medical surgeries or dermatology clinics.

Oral lichen planus is characterised by the presence of white patches which principally affect the buccal mucosa, lips, tongue and attached gingivae. Traditionally, lichen planus has been divided clinically into a number of subtypes, including reticular (fig. 17), erosive (fig. 18), plaque-like (fig. 19) and atrophic (fig. 20). However, such clear division is often difficult clinically and the mucosa of an individual patient may show evidence of different subtypes at different sites at any one time (fig. 21). In addition, subdivision of oral lichen planus has little influence on clinical management. Although the presence of lichen planus can be strongly

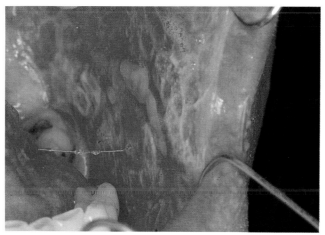

Fig. 21 Areas of reticular and erosive lichen planus affecting the buccal mucosa.

suspected clinically, especially in cases with accompanying skin involvement, it is advisable to confirm the diagnosis by mucosal biopsy when clinical doubt persists. Lichen planus is not a well defined clinical entity and therefore biopsy material should be taken from a typical affected area of mucosa and not from areas of erosion. In addition, when large areas of the mucosa are involved, a buccal biopsy is more likely to provide information that will confirm the clinical diagnosis than tissue taken from the tongue. Interestingly, palatal involvement is rare and, as a generalisation, patients with lesions which are clinically suggestive of lichen planus at this site are more likely to be suffering from a lichenoid reaction.

If the patient is asymptomatic, then no active treatment is required. However, a small percentage of patients suffer from discomfort, particularly when erosive areas develop. In these circumstances, topical steroid therapy such as hydrocortisone hemisuccinate (2·5 mg pellet) or betamethasone valerate (0·5 mg tablet) should be provided. The patient must be instructed to allow the steroid to dissolve adjacent to the lesion two to four times daily until clinical improvement occurs. Topical steroid therapy in the form of a cream or

ointment has also been suggested, but patients often find these preparations difficult to use and therefore likely to be of minimal benefit. The usual precautions concerning steroid therapy should be observed whenever systemic steroid therapy is contemplated for patients with lichen planus.

Griseofulvin (500 mg twice daily for 3 months) has been found to be helpful in patients with erosive lichen planus which fails to respond to topical steroid therapy. If griseofulvin is prescribed, then it is advisable to monitor liver function haematologically (10 ml clotted sample) and warn female patients using oral contraceptive drugs that additional precautions are essential due to reduced effectiveness of the oral contraceptive.

Lichenoid reactions
Lichenoid reactions may be clinically indistinguishable from lichen planus. However, asymmetry and involvement of the palate are suggestive of a lichenoid reaction rather than lichen planus. Patients suspected of having a lichenoid drug reaction will often give a history of drug therapy known to produce such white patches and this can be helpful in diagnosis.

8

Salivary gland disease

Conditions which affect salivary tissue may either be limited to one individual gland or may be present in all glands. Symptoms of salivary gland disease are therefore either localised to the glands themselves or result in reduced production of saliva. Investigations which may be undertaken in a clinical context and the value of specialist investigations are discussed in this chapter.

Salivary disorders are fairly common and can be divided clinically into those which affect the major glands (parotid, submandibular or sublingual) and those which arise in the minor glands. A surgical sieve approach to the diagnosis of salivary gland disease is helpful, since it classifies conditions into either congenital or acquired lesions, with the latter grouping being subdivided into infective, traumatic, neoplastic and miscellaneous.

Congenital disease

Developmental abnormalities of the salivary glands are extremely uncommon and will therefore rarely be encountered in dental practice. Although any developmental defect will have been present from birth, it may only be first noticed in early adolescence when advanced caries and periodontal disease, secondary to xerostomia, will become obvious (fig. 1).

Interestingly, developmental abnormalities of the major salivary glands are often accompanied by other defects such as absence of lacrimal glands and the eyes should therefore be examined for lack of tears. Confirmation of the absence of salivary gland tissue can be made using scintiscanning (fig. 2) or CT scanning. Unfortunately, once diagnosed there is little that can be offered in the way of treatment for such patients, although a high level of oral hygiene must be maintained and preventive measures, including dietary advice, instituted. Clearly, any opportunistic infections, in particular candidosis, should be treated promptly.

Infective disease
Viral infection
A variety of viruses, including paramyxovirus, echovirus, coxsackie group, influenza, parainfluenza and Epstein-Barr, can affect the major salivary glands. Patients may show a degree of systemic upset, but this is variable and some individuals may have had asymptomatic infection.

The paramyxovirus responsible for mumps has an incubation period of up to 3 weeks prior to the development of obvious salivary gland involvement. A characteristic feature of mumps is the development of painful parotid or submandibular swelling which is usually bilateral, although unilateral cases can occur (fig. 3). Clinical diagnosis can be confirmed by demonstrating significant antibody levels to S and V mumps antigens (10 ml clotted sample).

The mumps virus persists in saliva for about 10 days following the appearance of clinical signs and outbreaks therefore tend to occur in clusters since infection is transmitted by droplet spread. No effective treatment is available, but fortunately the outcome is usually uneventful, although a small number of adult patients may develop complications such as orchitis, oophoritis or meningoencephalitis. An episode of mumps confers lifelong immunity to further attacks, since the virus exists as one serological type. The incidence of mumps is decreasing in some countries, possibly owing to the introduction of active immunisation programmes.

Clinically, it may be impossible to differentiate mumps from the other viral infections which can affect the major salivary glands. Therefore, serological estimation of antibody levels are required for definitive diagnosis and these also provide useful epidemiological information. Infection with these less common viruses is a possible explanation for the fact that some patients believe that they have had mumps more than once. Again, no active treatment is required in those circumstances, but patient isolation will help reduce spread within the community.

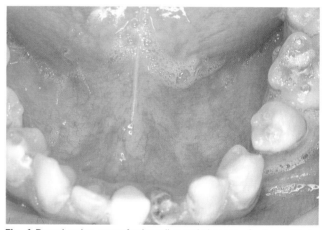

Fig. 1 Dental caries, scant frothy saliva and absence of submandibular duct papillae in a teenager with congenital absence of all major salivary glands.

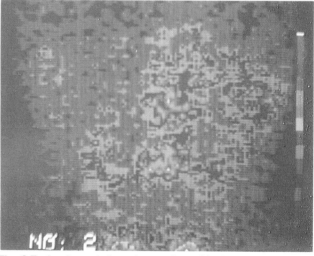

Fig. 2 Technetium scintiscan in a patient with absent major salivary glands. The lobes of the thyroid gland at the bottom of the picture take up isotope normally.

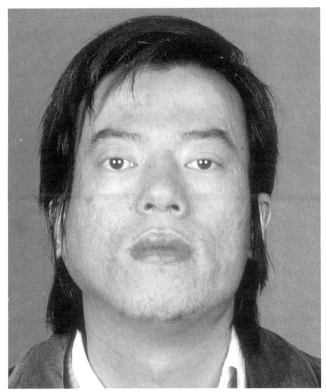

Fig. 3 Right parotid enlargement in a patient with mumps. (Reprinted by kind permission from: *Pocket picture guide, oral medicine*. London: Gower Medical Publishing, 1988).

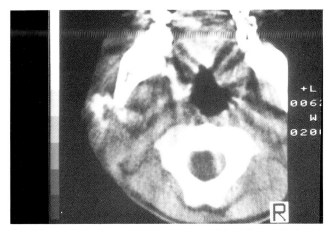

Fig. 4 Computerised tomographic sialogram of the left parotid gland in a child. The multiple filling defects were due to the caseation associated with tuberculous infection.

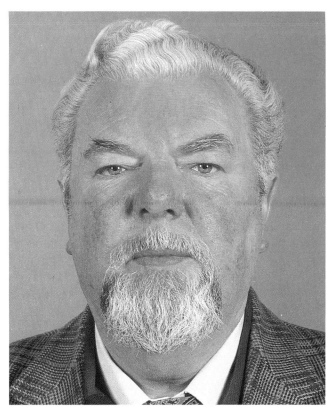

Fig. 5 Acute suppurative parotitis showing enlargement of the left parotid gland.

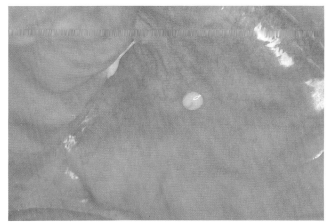

Fig. 6 Pus exuding from the left parotid gland orifice.

Bacterial infection

Bacterial infections of the salivary glands generally develop owing to spread of microorganisms from the oral flora along the excretory duct. An exception to this is tuberculosis which, although a rare disease, can spread by the haematogenous route into the major salivary glands (fig. 4).

In the past, suppurative parotitis was a common post-operative complication of major abdominal surgery, but the advent of antibiotics and a better understanding of fluid balance has now overcome this problem. However, although acute suppurative sialadenitis is now rarely seen in hospitalised patients, it is encountered relatively frequently in out-patients. Infection characteristically produces symptoms of pain and swelling in one gland (fig. 5). Cervical lymphadenopathy may also be present and intra-oral examination should reveal pus exuding from the affected gland orifice

(fig. 6). If infection is the result of duct obstruction due to the presence of a sialolith, then removal of the stone will achieve drainage and be followed by a copious flow of pus (fig. 7).

The management of acute suppurative sialadenitis involves obtaining a sample of pus (preferably as aspirate from the duct) which should be sent for culture and antibiotic sensitivity testing. Traditionally, the microorganisms encountered in acute bacterial sialadenitis have been streptococci and staphylococci. However, as has been found in other acute oral infections, it is becoming increasingly apparent that anaerobic bacteria are likely to play an important role. To date the vast majority of bacteria implicated in this infection have been found to be sensitive to a range of antibiotics. Unfortunately, definitive sensitivity information is rarely available within the first 48 hours and, therefore, choice of antibiotic therapy has to be made empirically. Our preferred regime is an initial single 3 g load of amoxycillin, followed by a dose of 250 mg 8-hourly for 5 days. Alternatively, erythromycin (250 mg 6-hourly may be used in patients with a known hypersensitivity to the penicillin group of antibiotics. Patients should be advised on the use of hot salt mouthwashes to encourage drainage and be provided, if necessary, with analgesics.

Sialography is indicated following resolution of an acute episode of sialadenitis, since the majority of even otherwise healthy individuals have some local but correctable gland abnormality, such as a benign stricture (fig. 8), mucous plug or sialolith. In the past, it was the failure to account and correct these local predisposing factors which meant that many patients suffered needlessly from recurrent episodes of infection. Concomitant diseases, such as Sjögren's syndrome or previous radiotherapy to the head and neck, will also predispose to the development of acute bacterial sialadenitis and the presence of these factors should be noted.

A specific parotid disease of a non-obstructive nature occurs in children and is known as chronic recurrent parotitis of childhood (CRPC). Prior to diagnosis, a child with CRPC will characteristically suffer from multiple episodes of parotitis, which are usually treated empirically with antibiotics. However, if sialography is performed in a quiescent phase of the disease, it will reveal sialectasis, a diagnostic feature of CRPC (fig. 9). Surprisingly, although sialectasis may be demonstrated in both glands, each episode of infection tends to affect only one side. It is generally accepted that CRPC resolves around puberty and, interestingly, the sialographic features can return to normal as the patient becomes older. At the present time, treatment options for CRPC appear to be based on either providing antibiotic therapy when each episode occurs, or providing the child with long-term prophylactic antibiotics. Our own experience would support a long-term antibiotic regime since it is likely to minimise the risk of permanent gland damage.

A specific diagnostic problem can occur when a child presents with a painless swelling along the lower border of the jaw which could be either salivary or dental in origin. If clinical examination, including radiographs, fails to reveal dental disease, and bimanual palpation of the submandibular gland is painless with expression of clear saliva, then the child may well be suffering from staphylococcal lymphadenitis (fig. 10). This rare condition is thought to arise due to spread of staphylococcal infection from a nasopharyngeal focus. The absence of any systemic upset, including pyrexia, in such cases is characteristic and if diagnosed then erythromycin or flucloxacillin therapy should be instituted.

Discussion of salivary gland infection must include mention of rare conditions such as actinomycosis, gonorrhoea and cat scratch disease, all of which can affect the major salivary glands. Infection of the minor glands due to *Mycoplasma pneumoniae* has been reported and can produce a transient labial gland enlargement.

Traumatic disease
Under this heading it is proposed to discuss three conditions, two (mucocele and ranula) which are almost certainly of traumatic origin and one (necrotising sialometaplasia) which may have trauma as an aetiological factor.

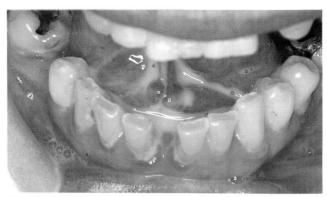
Fig. 7 Pus exuding into the floor of mouth from the left submandibular orifice immediately after removal of a sialolith.

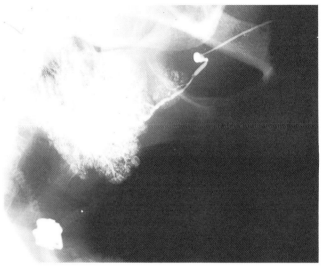
Fig. 8 Parotid sialogram showing a narrowing of the main duct approximately 2 cm from the parotid orifice.

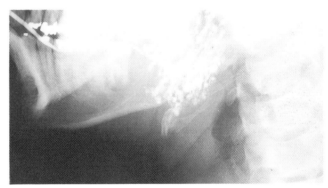
Fig. 9 Sialectasis in the parotid gland in a patient with chronic recurrent parotitis of childhood.

Mucocele
Trauma to an excretory duct may produce a collection of saliva, initially within the duct itself (mucus retention) and subsequently in the submucosal tissue (mucus extravasation). This lesion particularly affects the lower lip (fig. 11), but can arise at any intra-oral site where minor glands are situated. In children it has been suggested that trauma from erupting lower permanent incisors can predispose to the development of a mucocele on the ventral aspect of the tongue (fig. 12). Owing to the superficial nature of most mucoceles, they often discharge spontaneously within 24–48 hours, although recurrence is common. In view of this, patients characteristically present with a complaint of a recurring 'blister' rather than a persistent swelling.

41

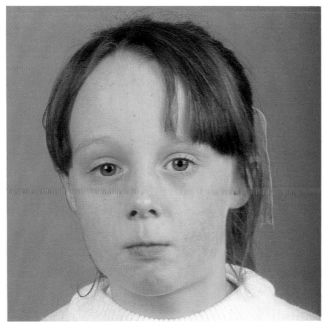

Fig. 10 Typical presentation of staphylococcal lymphadenitis of childhood.

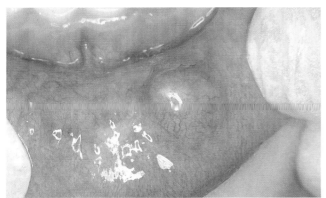

Fig. 11 Mucocele arising from a minor salivary gland in the lower lip.

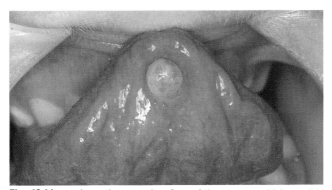

Fig. 12 Mucocele on the ventral surface of the tongue, which possibly arose as a result of trauma from erupting incisor teeth.

The treatment of a mucocele consists of surgical removal of the 'cyst' along with the affected salivary tissue. Incision of the overlying mucosa, followed by careful blunt dissection, will usually permit removal of the lesion intact and limit damage to the adjacent structures, in particular blood vessels and nerves. Although rare, post-operative complications can occur and the patient should be warned pre-operatively of the risk of bruising or transient nerve paraesthesia. Some specialists advocate cryotherapy as an alternative to the surgical treatment of mucoceles.

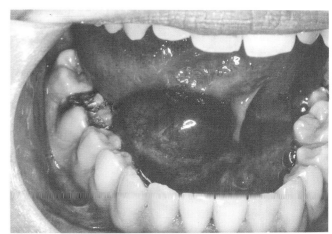

Fig. 13 Ranula arising in the right sublingual gland.

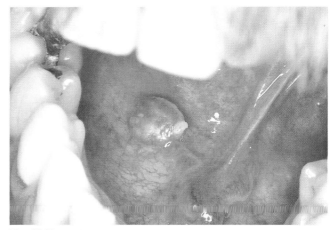

Fig. 14 Mucocele overlying the right sublingual gland.

Ranula
A ranula is a form of mucocele which arises from one of the sublingual glands and typically presents as a large non-painful bluish swelling on one side of the floor of mouth (fig. 13). This should not be confused with a mucocele arising in a superficial minor gland in this region (fig. 14). Marsupialisation with packing is the treatment of choice for a ranula, since attempts at enucleation are likely to be unsuccessful owing to the friable and extensive nature of the cyst lining.

Necrotising sialometaplasia
Trauma has been speculated upon as playing a role in the development of necrotising sialometaplasia, which classically presents as an area of ulceration in the palate (fig. 15). Prior to the onset of ulceration, some patients have described episodes of anaesthesia or paraesthesia of the greater palatine nerve. In some cases there has been a history of recent palatal infiltration of local anaesthetic agent and this, combined with histological evidence of minor salivary infarction, has led to trauma being proposed as a possible aetiological factor. Necrotising sialometaplasia can resemble squamous cell carcinoma both clinically and histologically and, unfortunately, in the past some patients have undergone major resection for what in retrospect was found to be a benign condition. Necrotising sialometaplasia will resolve without treatment in 10–14 days and recurrence is rare.

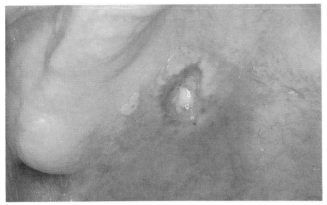

Fig. 15 Palatal ulcer which was painless and shown histologically to be necrotising sialometaplasia.

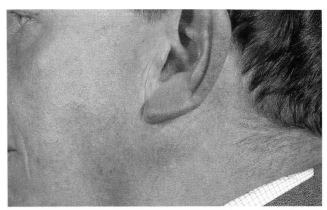

Fig. 16 Parotid gland enlargement due to pleomorphic salivary adenoma which had been present for 6 years. Note upward deflection of ear lobe.

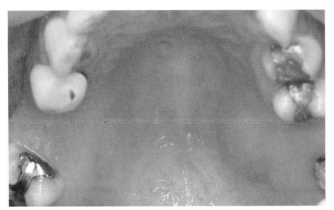

Fig. 17 Palatal swelling in the left first molar region, due to a mucoepidermoid salivary gland neoplasm.

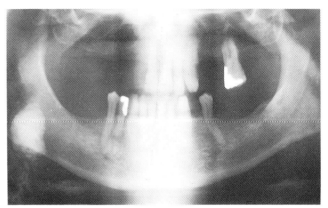

Fig. 18 A dental panoramic tomograph showing a large radiopacity in the region of the right submandibular gland. Sialography confirmed this to be an intraglandular sialolith.

Neoplastic disease

Pleomorphic salivary adenoma accounts for the majority (around 80%) of tumours in the parotid gland (fig. 16), whilst in the submandibular gland a relatively high proportion (60%) of lesions are either adenoid cystic carcinoma, mucoepidermoid tumour or adenocarcinoma. Neoplasms of the sublingual salivary gland are virtually all malignant, whilst in the minor salivary glands around 50% of lesions are malignant. Interestingly, the majority of minor gland tumours occur in the palate (fig. 17) or upper lip and therefore, from a practical point of view, whilst a localised swelling of the lower lip is likely to be a mucocele, a similar swelling of the upper lip could well represent the presence of malignancy.

Clearly, any lesion suspected of being a salivary gland neoplasm requires early biopsy. Once diagnosed then other appropriate investigations, such as sialography, CT scanning or magnetic resonance imaging are helpful in determining the extent of the tumour. A clinical feature suggestive of malignancy within the parotid gland is facial nerve weakness or palsy, and in this context it is important to recall that carcinomatous change can occur within a pre-existing benign condition (carcinoma ex-pleomorphic salivary adenoma).

Miscellaneous diseases

A variety of salivary disorders of diverse aetiology including salivary gland calculus, drug-induced disease, Sjögren's syndrome, xerostomia and sialorrhoea are considered under this heading.

Salivary calculus (sialolith)

Calcified deposits known as salivary calculi or sialoliths may develop in any of the salivary glands. In the parotid gland they are virtually always present in the duct itself, whereas in the submandibular gland they may be found either in the duct or within the gland (fig. 18). Characteristically, the presence of salivary calculus initially produces transient episodes (1–2 hours) of gland swelling, particularly at meal-times. The development of such swellings is usually associated with mild discomfort, although at the time of examination there may be no clinical abnormality. Since approximately 20% of salivary calculi are radiopaque, they will not always be detected in routine radiographs, although all should be apparent on sialographic views.

Treatment is based on surgical removal (fig. 19), which is relatively easy when the calculus is placed at the duct orifice or in the anterior part of the duct. When the submandibular gland is affected, temporary sutures should initially be placed distal to the calculus, to prevent any distal displacement during removal. Once removed, attempts at primary closure of the duct may result in the formation of strictures and it is therefore best to leave the wound open rather than attempt primary closure. If the lesion is intraglandular then no active treatment may be undertaken, but with time partial gland obstruction will almost certainly lead to recurrent episodes of acute bacterial sialadenitis. In these circumstances, therefore, removal of the gland has to be considered.

Minor salivary gland calculi do occur, but are generally asymptomatic and only observed as an incidental histological finding.

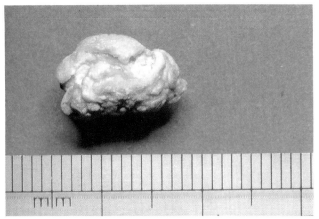

Fig. 19 Sialolith which was excised from a submandibular gland duct.

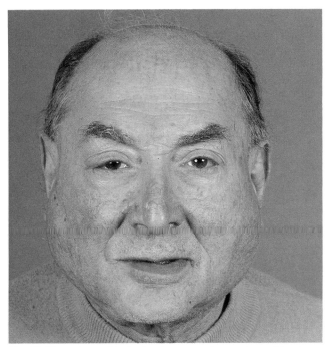

Fig. 20 Bilateral parotid gland enlargement in a patient with primary Sjögren's syndrome.

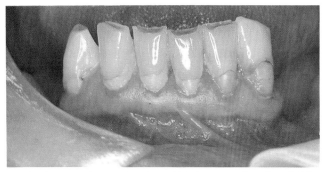

Fig. 21 Pattern of cervical caries which is suggestive of underlying xerostomia.

Drug-induced disease

Antihypertensive agents, or those with an anticholinergic activity, such as tricyclic antidepressants, tend to decrease salivary gland flow, leading to the complaint of xerostomia. In contrast to this, benzodiazepines may produce increased salivary flow in children or the elderly. The mechanism by which drugs alter salivary flow is uncertain, although in the case of overuse of diuretics the xerostomia produced is likely to be secondary to dehydration. In drug-induced xerostomia, the salivary glands are normal since it is a functional disorder and, therefore, a labial gland biopsy will not reveal any abnormality. When a drug is thought to be responsible for altered salivary production, then it may be possible, in liaison with the patient's doctor or physician, to consider alternative therapy.

Sjögren's syndrome

Sjögren's syndrome is currently the subject of much research worldwide. Two variants which are possibly distinct types are recognised: primary Sjögren's (previously known as Sicca syndrome) involves dry eyes/dry mouth whilst in secondary Sjögren's syndrome (previously known as Sjögren's syndrome) an autoimmune disorder, usually a connective tissue disease, is present in addition to dry eyes and/or dry mouth. Parotid gland enlargement is clinically obvious in approximately 15% of patients (fig. 20), but is also reported by a further 15% of patients. Rarely, lacrimal gland enlargement and cranial nerve lesions may also occur, the latter feature being particularly associated with patients who have systemic lupus erythematosus.

Both types of Sjögren's syndrome principally occur in the elderly population, with females being affected more commonly than males. A range of disorders are associated with secondary Sjögren's syndrome, including primary biliary cirrhosis, rheumatoid arthritis, systemic lupus erythematosus and systemic sclerosis. The major oral component of Sjögren's syndrome is xerostomia which predisposes to a number of dental problems (fig. 21). The oral mucosa will usually appear dry and a lobulated appearance of the dorsal surface of the tongue is a common feature (fig. 22).

It is generally accepted that labial gland biopsy is the most useful investigation to confirm the presence of Sjögren's syndrome. This investigation is simple and quick to perform, since numerous labial glands are present beneath the mucosa of the lower lip. Incision of the labial mucosa in the canine region permits removal of at least five lobules of salivary gland tissue. As with removal of mucoceles at the site, patients should be warned of the risk of temporary paraesthesia or bruising in the mental region following surgery.

The management of the oral component of Sjögren's syndrome involves vigorous treatment of the xerostomia (see xerostomia below). Trials of systemic drug therapy which attempt to increase salivary gland function in Sjögren's patients are ongoing and claims have already been made for the efficacy of evening oil of primrose. Recently, a combined professional and patient self-help group, termed the British Sjögren's Syndrome Association, has been formed and will provide further information and membership forms on request (see p43).

Xerostomia

It has been reported that, when questioned, as many as 10% of unselected patients will report that they suffer from a dry mouth, although the majority of these individuals are likely to have normal salivary gland function. A true reduction in salivary function can be either due to primary gland disease, such as Sjögren's syndrome, or post-operative radiation damage, or be a secondary phenomenon of anxiety, dehydration or drug therapy.

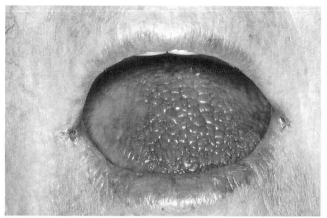

Fig. 22 Obvious xerostomia and a lobulated appearance to the tongue in a patient with Sjögren's syndrome. The angular cheilitis was secondary to oral candidosis.

Patients who suffer from a prolonged reduction of saliva are likely to complain of difficulty in swallowing and talking, altered taste and, if worn, poor retention of their dentures. Reduced levels of saliva will also predispose to opportunistic oral infections, particularly candidosis, and lead to an increase in periodontal disease and caries.

Clinical examination of healthy patients should reveal saliva pooling in the floor of the mouth, whereas if xerostomia is present the amount of saliva is not only reduced but may also appear frothy. A useful test is to place a mirror against the buccal mucosa and this should lift off easily when saliva is present in normal amounts. Degrees of stickiness during this manoeuvre is a useful indication of reduced saliva production. Each of the major glands should be palpated and clear saliva seen to be expressed from each duct orifice. Unstimulated and stimulated flow rates may be obtained from individual major or minor glands, but this requires specialist equipment and is not likely to be practical in general dental practice.

Treatment of patients with xerostomia is based on achieving adequate levels of saliva in the mouth by the use of artificial saliva substitutes, such as Saliva Orthana, Luborant and Glandosane. The first two substitutes come in hand-held pump-action dispensers. Glandosane, however, has an aerosol propellent and has the potential disadvantage in dentate individuals of predisposing to enamel demineralisation. In addition, intensive preventive measures should be instituted in dentate individuals along with prompt treatment of oral candidosis or bacterial salivary gland infection. The design of any dentures should be optimised in edentulous individuals in order to minimise trauma of the atrophic oral mucosa.

Sialorrhoea

The complaint of excess salivation is considerably less common than the complaint of xerostomia. In sialorrhoea, patients complain of 'saliva continually drooling out of their mouths', 'having to dab the angles of their mouths all the time' or 'waking up at night with the pillow soaked in saliva'. Increased salivation is a recognised problem in patients who have diabetic autonomic neuropathy, Parkinson's disease, cerebral palsy or difficulty in adapting to new dentures. In these circumstances, incoordination or reduced swallowing rate may also, in part, be contributing to the complaint of excess salivation. In the absence of any organic basis to their complaint, patients who complain of sialorrhoea are usually not psychologically normal, although the exact basis of their abnormality is as yet ill-defined.

In the past, the provision of hyoscyamine sulphate (0·2 mg, two to three times daily) has been helpful in alleviating the symptoms of sialorrhoea, but unfortunately this drug has now been discontinued and there are no reliable alternatives at present.

Sjögren's Syndrome: The British Sjögren's Syndrome Association, c/o Joan Patel, 7 Winchdells, Bennetts End, Hemel Hempstead HP3 8HZ.

Saliva Orthana: A. S. Orthana Kemisk, Fabrik 35 Englandsvej, DK-2770, Kastrup, Copenhangen, Denmark, and Nycomed (UK) Ltd, 2111 Coventry Road, Sheldon, Birmingham B26 3EA.

Glandosane: Fresenius AG, D-6380, Bad Homburg, FRG. Distributed by Fresenius Ltd, 6-7 Christleton Court, Stuart Road, Manor Park, Runcorn, Cheshire.

Luborant: Antigen Ltd, Dublin, Ireland. Distributed by Antigen International Ltd, Runcorn, Cheshire.

9

Dermatoses and pigmentary disorders

This chapter considers the presentation, diagnosis and treatment of dermatological disorders which may affect the oral mucosa, either alone or in combination with cutaneous lesions. Although the majority of mucocutaneous disorders are associated with minimal symptoms, some may cause considerable morbidity. Diagnosis of pigmentary changes of the oral mucosa is also considered.

In view of the developmental similarity between skin and the oral mucosa, it is not surprising that pathological conditions may occur simultaneously at both sites. Indeed, a number of mucocutaneous disorders may initially present with oral lesions and the dental surgeon therefore has a key role to play in early diagnosis.

Lichen planus/lichenoid reactions

Lichen planus and lichenoid reactions, two disorders which frequently affect the oral mucosa, have been discussed earlier, in the chapters on white patches and orofacial allergic reactions. However, in both conditions the oral lesions can also be accompanied by cutaneous involvement. Skin lesions of lichen planus are characteristically described as dusky pink papules and are commonly found on the wrists, forearms and legs (fig. 1). The appearance of drug-induced cutaneous lichenoid reactions is variable but may present as erythematous areas of skin at any site (fig. 2). Occasionally, systemic administration of a drug produces cutaneous changes (a so-called fixed drug eruption) at the same site on each occasion it is given (fig. 3).

Pemphigus

Pemphigus is an uncommon vesiculobullous disorder which occurs in four forms: pemphigus vulgaris, pemphigus foliaceous, pemphigus vegitans and pemphigus erythematosus. Pemphigus vulgaris is the most frequently encountered form and classically affects the middle-aged or elderly patient, although rare cases have been reported in childhood and adolescence. The clinical onset of pemphigus is insidious, developing over several weeks and, interestingly, approximately half of the cases first present with oral lesions (fig. 4). The initial features may be linked to non-specific mucosal erosions, although these are soon accompanied by cutaneous changes. Confirmation of the clinical diagnosis is based on histopathological examination, preferably accompanied by immunofluorescent investigations on frozen tissue.

Unfortunately, it is not possible to predict which individuals with pemphigus will develop extensive skin involvement (fig. 5), with the associated risk of rapid alterations of protein and electrolyte balance. Therefore, whenever pemphigus is diagnosed the patient requires immediate hospitalisation. In the past pemphigus was fatal,

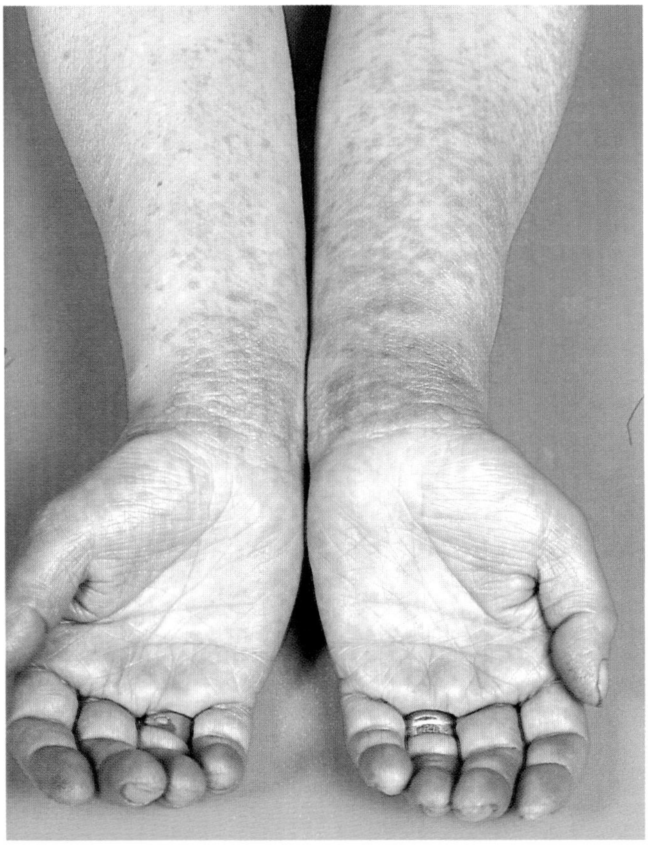

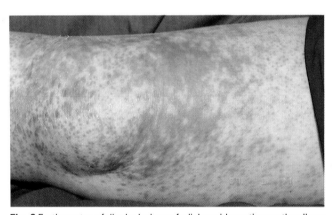

Fig. 2 Erythematous folicular lesions of a lichenoid reaction on the elbow (courtesy of Dr N. B. Simpson, Glasgow Royal Infirmary).

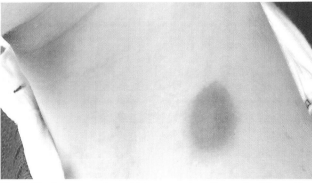

Fig. 3 Fixed drug eruption which occurred on the neck of the patient each time she was given co-trimoxazole.

Fig. 1 Papular lesions of cutaneous lichen planus affecting the wrists and forearms.

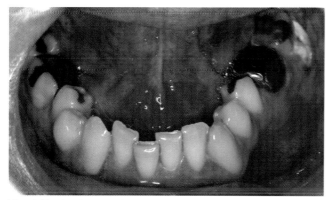

Fig. 4 Erosive lesions of pemphigus in the floor of the mouth and attached gingivae in the lower left molar region.

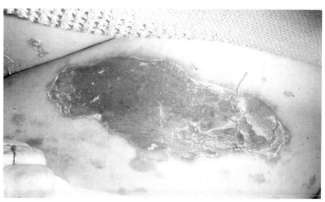

Fig. 5 Extensive cutaneous lesions of pemphigus (courtesy of Dr N. B. Simpson, Glasgow Royal Infirmary).

but with the advent of potent systemic corticosteroid therapy, prognosis has been dramatically improved. Treatment is now based on the institution of high-dose prednisolone (50–100 mg daily) to bring the disease under control. Once control is established, patients can be maintained on a steroid dose of approximately 20 mg of prednisolone daily. Use of the immunomodulatory drug azathioprine (50–100 mg) daily can also be considered since this has the advantage of allowing the amount of steroid therapy to be further reduced. Indirect immunofluorescence is helpful in monitoring the effectiveness of treatment since the serum titre of intra-epithelial IgG reflects the degree of disease activity.

Pemphigoid

As a generalisation, two forms of pemphigoid are recognised: bullous pemphigoid and mucous membrane pemphigoid. In bullous pemphigoid, cutaneous lesions dominate the clinical picture whilst in mucous membrane pemphigoid cutaneous lesions occur infrequently. The oral features of mucous membrane pemphigoid are non-specific but often involve irregular areas of ulceration (fig. 6) or desquamative gingivitis (fig. 7). Histopathological examination of the mucosa of a patient with pemphigoid will reveal a subepithelial split and direct immunofluorescence will show deposition of IgG and complement in the basal region.

Treatment of pemphigoid is based on the use of topical steroid preparations, such as betamethasone lozenges or hydrocortisone pellets, although systemic therapy may be required in severe cases. When there is extensive oral involvement cyclophosphamide, in conjunction with steroids, may be helpful. Fluocinolone acetonide cream applied to the tissues using extended vacuum-formed splints and held in place for 5 minutes in the morning and for 5 minutes in the evening for 6 weeks has been found to be useful in the management of desquamative lesions of the gingivae (fig. 8).

It is important that all patients who have been diagnosed as having mucous membrane pemphigoid receive a consultant ophthalmic opinion, since ocular lesions can accompany the disease. The ophthalmologist will be looking primarily for symblepharon (fig. 9), although there may also be an association between mucous membrane pemphigoid and glaucoma. If genital lesions occur, then the patient should also be referred to the appropriate specialist.

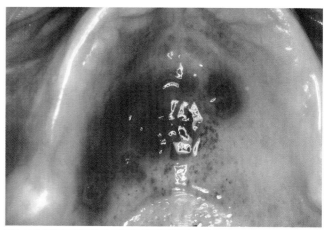

Fig. 6 Palatal lesions of mucous membrane pemphigoid.

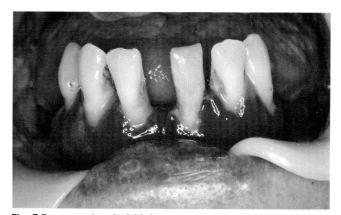

Fig. 7 Desquamative gingivitis in mucous membrane pemphigoid.

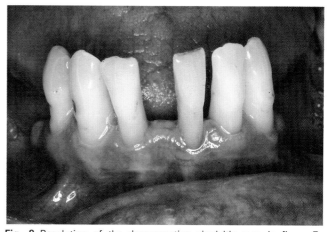

Fig. 8 Resolution of the desquamative gingivitis seen in figure 7, following topical fluocinolone acetonide therapy.

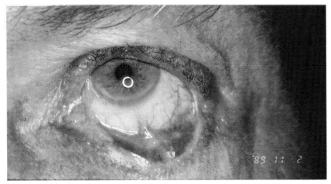

Fig. 9 Ocular involvement in mucous membrane pemphigoid.

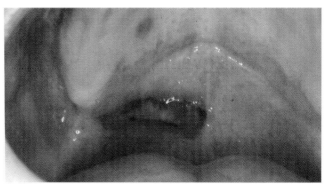

Fig. 10 Recently ruptured bulla of angina bullosa haemorrhagica in the palate.

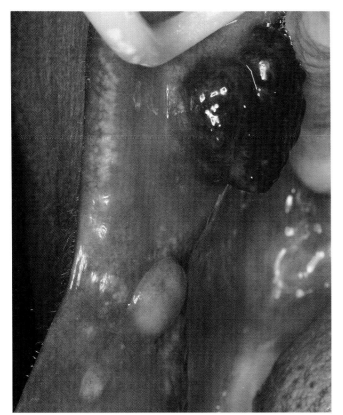

Fig. 11 Blood-filled bulla which developed as a consequence of thrombocytopenia in a leukaemic patient.

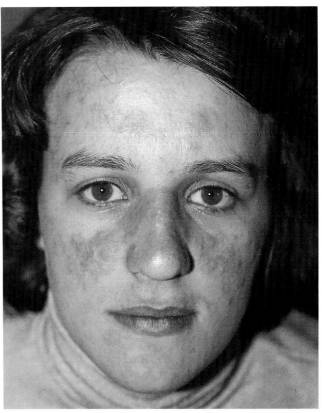

Fig. 12 Characteristic facial appearance (butterfly rash) of a patient with SLE.

Angina bullosa haemorrhagica

The term angina bullosa haemorrhagica (ABH) was originally used to describe recurrent intra-oral blood blisters. The clinical history of such patients is remarkably uniform and involves the complaint of a solitary blister which develops within seconds or minutes, usually on the soft palate during eating, although in some cases the blister arises spontaneously. The lesions can be sufficiently large to cause a sensation of choking, and the patient will therefore often deliberately burst the blister.

Alternatively, some patients are so alarmed by the condition that they seek treatment at their local accident and emergency department. If left untreated the blister will usually burst spontaneously within 24 hours, leaving an ulcerated area surrounded by evidence of haemorrhage (fig. 10). The pathological basis of ABH is unknown, but it has been claimed that a history of steroid therapy, either given systemically or in the form of an inhaler, may be a predisposing factor. Histopathological examination of an intact, blood-filled blister reveals features identical to mucous membrane pemphigoid, but immunofluorescence is negative in ABH.

No active treatment other than reassurance is required. Total resolution of the lesion usually occurs within 7–10 days. Generally, patients with ABH suffer 5–10 episodes over 2–3 years, and the condition then remits spontaneously. If the history is not classical of ABH then a full blood count to exclude thrombocytopenia is mandatory for patients presenting with a blood-filled bulla (fig. 11).

Lupus erythematosus

Lupus erythematosus occurs in two forms, either systemic or discoid. Systemic lupus erythematosus (SLE) usually occurs in women under 30 years of age and can affect most systems of the body, including skin (fig. 12), kidney, brain and salivary tissue. When the salivary glands are affected, SLE forms the

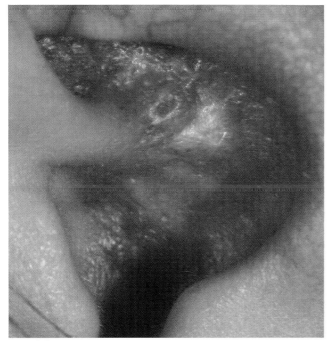

Fig. 13 Characteristic scarring lesions of DLE in the outer ear.

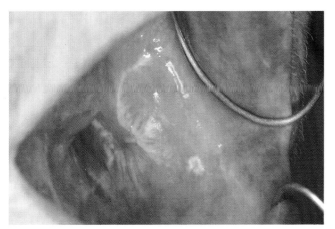

Fig. 14 Mucosal involvement in systemic lupus erythematosus.

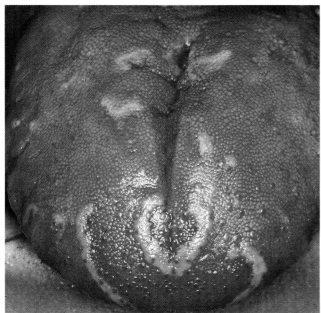

Fig. 15 Classical geographic tongue.

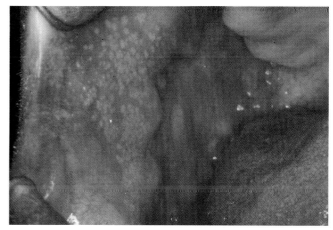

Fig. 16 Numerous sebaceous glands (Fordyce spots), occurring in the buccal mucosa.

connective tissue component of Sjögren's syndrome. Almost all patients with SLE have high titres of circulating antinuclear factor and if this is detected then referral to an appropriate physician is indicated.

Discoid lupus erythematosus (DLE) is also more common in women than men, and tends to occur in the third or fourth decade. Any area of skin may be involved, although lesions are more common in the ear (fig. 13) and areas which are exposed to sunlight. Oral lesions consisting of white patches which resemble lichen planus both clinically and histologically may occur in either form of lupus erythematosus (fig. 14). Treatment of oral lesions is symptomatic and involves the use of topical steroid preparations.

Other dermatoses

Of the other dermatoses which can affect the oral cavity, white sponge naevus and erythema multiforme have already been discussed in previous chapters. Dermatoses such as linear IgA disease, epidermolysis bullosa acquisita and dermatitis herpetiformis can have oral lesions, but these conditions are rare and will not be described here. However, it has been suggested that psoriasis, which is one of the commonest skin conditions seen in dermatology clinics in the UK, is related to the development of geographic tongue (fig. 15). Interestingly, psoriasis and geographic tongue have a similar histological appearance and it has been claimed that geographic tongue occurs particularly frequently in the guttate form of psoriasis. Geographic tongue may either be asymptomatic or produce a complaint of discomfort on eating hot or spicy foods. It has recently been shown that some patients with geographic tongue have low levels of serum zinc and symptomatic geographic tongue appears to respond to systemic zinc therapy. The treatment of choice is a dispersible form of zinc (Solvazinc, Thames Laboratories) at a dose of 200 mg 8-hourly for 3 months.

Ectopic sebaceous glands

Ectopic sebaceous glands (Fordyce spots), which probably occur in the oral mucosa of most individuals, may sometimes be mistaken for mucosal disease. This is particularly true if the glands occur in very large numbers on the buccal mucosa or lips (fig. 16). In addition, sebaceous glands appear to become more prominent in later life and may cause concern in elderly patients who become worried that they represent

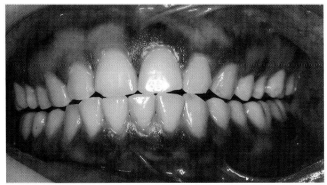

Fig. 17 Physiological pigmentation of gingivae.

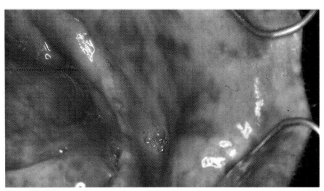

Fig. 18 Diffuse pigmentation of the buccal mucosa in a patient with Addison's disease.

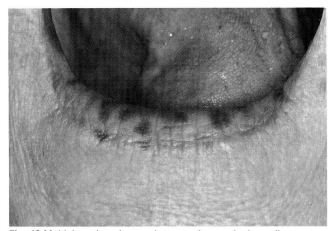

Fig. 19 Multiple melanotic macules occurring on the lower lip.

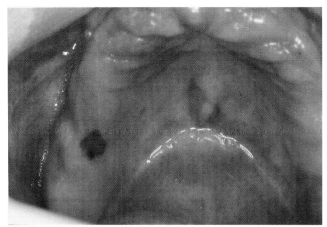

Fig. 20 Malignant melanoma on the upper edentulous ridge in a patient who had multiple areas of lentiginous change.

oral cancer. However, the clinical appearance is sufficiently characteristic that no active treatment is required other than reassurance of the benign nature of these glands.

Pigmentary disorders

Pigmentary changes which occur in the oral mucosa may be due to a number of conditions. Racial skin pigmentation is, as expected, often accompanied by mucosal pigmentation, although intra-oral pigmentation is also seen in approximately 15% of caucasians. Such mucosal pigmentation is usually diffuse but often involves the gingivae (fig. 17) or buccal mucosa. Increased melanin production may be stimulated by endocrine disturbances, in particular Addison's disease (fig. 18) or drugs such as oral contraceptives, antimalarials or tranquillisers. In addition, one of the most common causes of increased melanocyte activity in the oral cavity is smoking, which can produce diffuse pigmentation in the soft palate, buccal mucosa and the floor of the mouth. Melanotic macules may present as single or multiple lesions on the oral mucosa or lips (fig. 19). Such lesions are relatively common and do not require active treatment, unless they present an aesthetic problem to the patient. Biopsy is mandatory, however, to exclude the presence of malignant melanoma. Malignant melanoma is rare in the oral cavity, but when it does occur it is usually seen in the palate (fig. 20). Unfortunately, despite radical surgery the prognosis of intra-oral malignant melanoma is still very poor. Rarer causes of oral or peri-oral pigmentation include Peutz-Jegher's syndrome (fig. 21), Nelson's syndrome, fibrous dysplasia and HIV infection (fig. 22).

A discrete area of mucosal pigmentation known as an amalgam tattoo can be caused by accidental introduction of

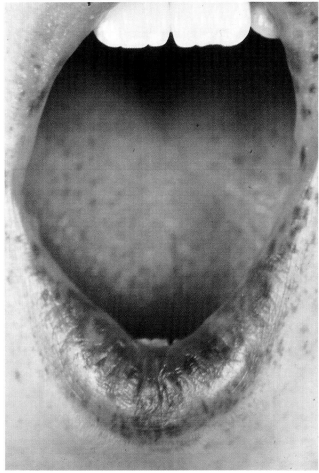

Fig. 21 Peri-oral lesions of Peutz-Jegher's syndrome.

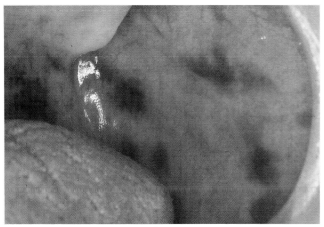

Fig. 22 Buccal pigmentation occurring in a patient with HIV infection.

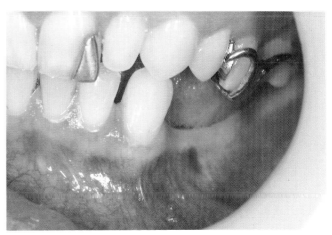

Fig. 23 Amalgam tattoo in the lower left premolar region.

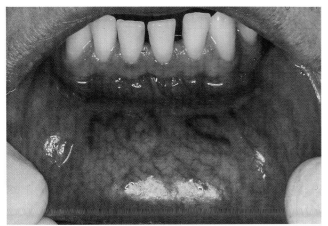

Fig. 24 Tattoo (Mick) on the lower lip of a patient called Martin!

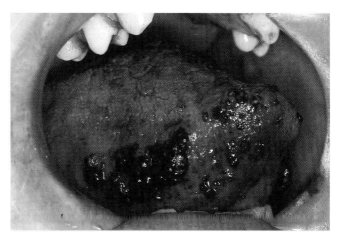

Fig. 25 Multiple haemangiomata within the tongue.

amalgam from dental restorations into the tissues, usually at the time of cavity preparation, tooth extraction or placement of retrograde root fillings (fig. 23). Tattoos may also be deliberately produced and patients have presented with names or other words tattooed on their oral mucosa (fig. 24).

The vascular abnormality, haemangioma, is relatively common intra-orally and can appear as a pigmented area of mucosa. The lesion is usually solitary, but may sometimes appear at multiple sites (fig. 25). Since the vascular nature of haemangioma is easily demonstrated clinically, diagnosis is straightforward. The majority of lesions are symptomless and require no treatment. However, if surgical removal is considered, this should be undertaken by a specialist surgeon in a hospital setting, owing to the risk of severe haemorrhage. Other treatment options which have been used include cryosurgery, arterial embolisation and injections of sclerosing agents.

10

The medically compromised patient

The following chapter describes the dental aspects of some of the more frequently occurring medical conditions which may have implications for dental treatment. Oral changes are often the first sign of the presence of systemic disease and the dental surgeon therefore has an important role to play in their early detection. In addition, it is essential to maintain oral health in patients who have systemic disorders which either limit their ability to carry out oral hygiene or are associated with a high incidence of mucosal and dental disease.

The definition of 'medically compromised' is somewhat arbitrary, but it can be interpreted as indicating the presence of a medical factor which may have implications for the provision of dental treatment. Although a wide spectrum of illnesses or drugs may affect patient management, it is only possible to cover the commoner ones in this article. In addition, it is not possible to discuss any implications which systemic disease or drug therapy may have for general anaesthesia.

Endocrine disorders

Two common endocrine conditions which involve altered hormonal levels are diabetes and pregnancy. Hormonal levels may also be affected as a result of the therapeutic use of corticosteroids.

Diabetes mellitus

Diabetes mellitus can present either in childhood (Type 1 or juvenile-onset diabetes) or in adulthood (Type 2 or maturity-onset diabetes). Although several disease processes can cause diabetes mellitus, it is generally agreed that in Type 1 diabetes there is an absolute deficiency of insulin, whereas in Type 2 diabetes there is a relative deficiency. Therefore treatment of Type 1 diabetes consists of provision of exogenous insulin by injection, whereas in Type 2 diabetes management usually involves reducing the patient's weight or increasing the tissue uptake of glucose by the use of oral hypoglycaemic agents. Only those diabetic patients who receive insulin can become hypoglycaemic. Hypoglycaemia can cause a collapse which must be treated urgently by the administration of either 10 g of glucose (two teaspoons of sugar or one third of a pint of milk) if the patient is conscious or 20 ml of 50% dextrose intravenously if the patient is unconscious. If glucose cannot be administered by either of these routes then glucagon (1 mg) can be given intramuscularly. A blood sample (2·5 ml in a yellow fluoride bottle) should be taken prior to the provision of glucose in order to assess the level of glucose at the time of collapse. Generally, any insulin-dependent diabetic should have an appointment first thing in the morning since glycaemic control should be optimal at this time because the patient will have recently taken his/her medication along with food.

There are no specific oral signs of diabetes mellitus, although a number of studies have described an increased incidence of caries and periodontal disease. Interestingly, it would also appear that oral candidosis is more common in diabetic patients and they also have clinical signs of infection at lower candidal loads than non-diabetics (fig. 1). One

possible reason for increased susceptibility to infection is the fact that candidal organisms are more adherent to the oral epithelium of diabetics and this adhesion is greater if glycaemic control is poor. Availability of carbohydrate in saliva may also be involved, since salivary glucose levels mirror blood glucose levels.

Management of a diabetic patient with intra-oral candidosis should take into account the type and quality of diabetes since the presence of poor glycaemic control is associated with difficulty in eradication of infection. Topical antifungal therapy, in the form of a nystatin pastille or amphotericin lozenge dissolved in the mouth four times daily, is effective in most cases, but it is essential that treatment is continued for at least 4 weeks. If infection persists beyond this time, then the use of a systemic antifungal drug, such as fluconazole or itraconazole, should be considered, following consultation with the patient's medical practitioner. Good denture hygiene should be encouraged and clearly there is a requirement for the patient to minimise carbohydrate intake. It has been claimed that xerostomia, which can predispose to oral candidosis, occurs frequently in diabetic patients, although at the present time this relationship is unproven since it has also been suggested that patients with

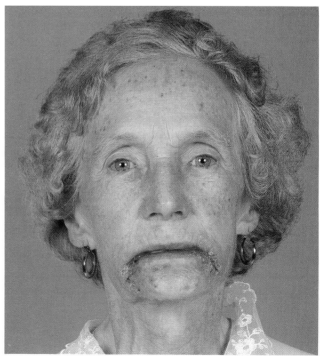

Fig. 1 Florid angular cheilitis due to candidal species in a patient with undiagnosed diabetes mellitus.

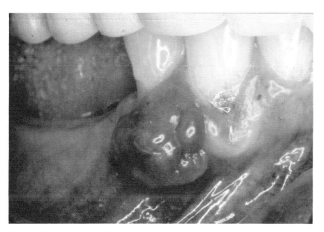

Fig. 2 Pregnancy epulis.

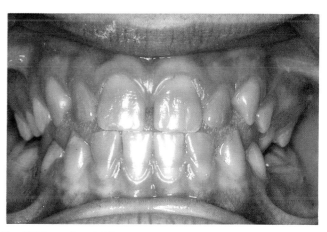

Fig. 3 Tetracycline staining.

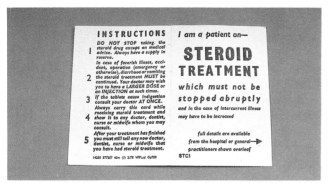

Fig. 4 Steroid warning card.

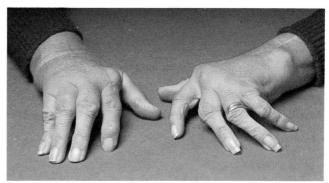

Fig. 5 Hands of a patient with severe rheumatoid arthritis.

longstanding diabetes mellitus produce more saliva than normal subjects.

Pregnancy

Pregnant women should not present any major problems during the provision of routine dental treatment under local anaesthesia, although in the third trimester the supine position should be avoided since it is likely to produce hypotension. A specific oral complication of pregnancy is the exacerbation of any pre-existing gingivitis and the development of localised gingival swellings (pregnancy epulis), which may appear at any time from the second month onwards (fig. 2). Any large lesions can be removed under local anaesthesia, but there is a risk of excessive haemorrhage, owing to the vascularity of the condition. If a surgical approach is used, then the patient should be warned that recurrence is likely although regression will occur soon after childbirth.

Radiography and the provision of systemic drug therapy should be limited during pregnancy, since it has implications for both mother and foetus. Tooth discolouration is a specific dental problem which can occur if any of the tetracyclines are taken during the time of tooth development (fig. 3). It is therefore sensible to avoid this group of antibiotics in pregnant women, women of childbearing age and children.

Corticosteroid therapy

Systemic corticosteroids are used to treat a number of medical conditions, but their use is associated with a variety of side-effects, most importantly adrenal suppression. Although adrenal suppression is more likely to occur when large amounts of steroid are given over a long period, it can develop after a course as short as 5 days. Any patient who is on or has received corticosteroid therapy within the previous 2 years should be regarded as having the potential for an adrenal crisis collapse if placed in a stressful situation. To avoid this problem a patient who is still receiving oral steroids can increase the dose on the day of treatment, whereas intravenous hydrocortisone (200 mg) can be administered immediately pre-operatively to those who have discontinued steroid therapy.

Steroid therapy can significantly worsen any infection, hypertension, diabetes or gastrointestinal ulceration the patient may have. Therefore great care has to be exercised in the therapeutic use of corticosteroid therapy and patients must be given a 'steroid warning card' giving details of the therapy prescribed (fig. 4).

Connective tissue disease

Rheumatoid arthritis (RA) is the commonest connective tissue disorder, with a typical onset between the ages of 30 and 40 years. Pain and swelling of the small joints of the hands and feet are a prominent early feature. RA may be associated with weakness of the ligaments in the neck and therefore careful neck support is required, especially during extractions, to prevent the serious risk of cervical dislocation. Severe involvement of joints in the legs will obviously restrict the patient's ability to attend the dental surgery, whilst hand lesions will limit the ability to maintain adequate oral hygiene (fig. 5). Iron deficiency frequently occurs in RA and this may also predispose the patient to recurrent aphthous stomatitis or candidal infection.

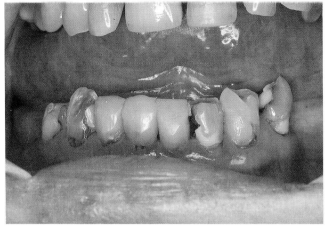

Fig. 6 Typical pattern of dental restorations and caries in a patient with Sjögren's syndrome.

When dry eyes or dry mouth occur along with a connective tissue disorder, then by definition the patient has secondary Sjögren's syndrome. Apart from an increased likelihood of dental caries (fig. 6), periodontal disease and salivary gland infections, patients with secondary Sjögren's syndrome may also develop mucosal changes as a side-effect of their anti-inflammatory drugs (fig. 7). In addition to mucosal lesions, taste abnormalities may also occur in patients receiving penicillamine therapy. Approximately 50% of RA patients with Sjögren's syndrome are allergic to antibiotics of the penicillin group and although the reasons for this are unknown it should be borne in mind when prescribing for bacterial infection or providing antibiotic prophylaxis for infective endocarditis.

Although the cause of systemic lupus erythematosus (SLE) is unknown, it is regarded as an auto-immune disease and is the second most common connective tissue component of secondary Sjögren's syndrome. The clinical presentation of lupus erythematosus is variable, but classically the disease affects women and involves fever, malaise, joint pains and a cutaneous rash (fig. 8). Approximately 20% of patients with SLE will at some time develop erosive white patches on the oral mucosa (fig. 9) which resemble lichen planus.

Systemic sclerosis (scleroderma) is an uncommon connective tissue disease which predominantly affects women. Unfortunately, the prognosis is poor and approximately 80% of sufferers have orofacial symptoms. Progressive changes in the tissues limit mouth opening and produce a 'pinched' or 'drawn' appearance to the face (fig. 10). Apart from the obvious problems of maintaining oral hygiene, patients with systemic sclerosis may also develop Sjögren's syndrome.

Cardiovascular disease
Three common cardiovascular conditions are hypertension, angina and myocardial infarction.

Hypertension
Hypertension may have no apparent cause (primary), or may be secondary to other conditions, in particular renal disease. The severity of the hypertension is likely to determine the type of treatment the patient will be given. Normally, patients are initially provided with diuretic therapy, but if this does not reduce the blood pressure sufficiently then the use of beta-blocker therapy, either alone or in combination with a diuretic

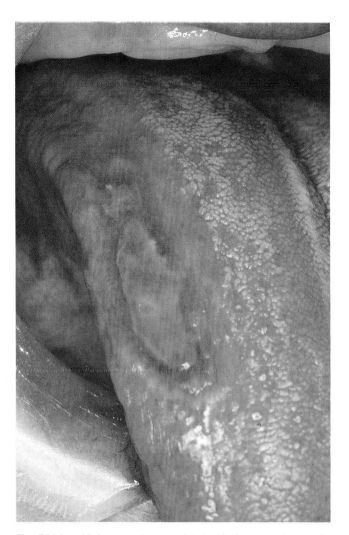

Fig. 7 Lichenoid drug reaction associated with the systemic use of a non-steroidal anti-inflammatory agent.

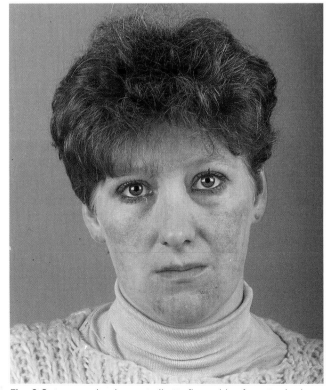

Fig. 8 Cutaneous involvement (butterfly rash) of systemic lupus erythematosus.

55

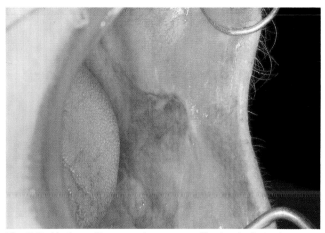

Fig. 9 Oral lesions of lupus erythematosus affecting the buccal mucosa.

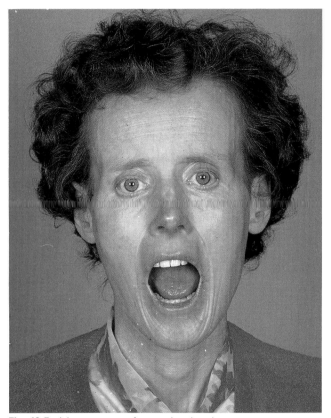

Fig. 10 Facial appearance of systemic sclerosis.

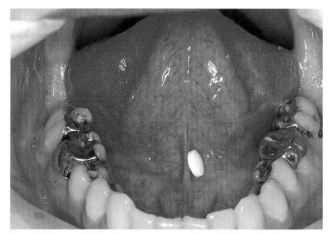

Fig. 11 Glyceryl trinitrate tablet placed sublingually for relief of an angina attack.

or a calcium channel blocking agent can be instituted. Hypertension in itself does not contra-indicate routine dental treatment but the drugs used to treat hypertension can cause a variety of oral problems, including xerostomia and lichenoid reactions. It is also recognised that nifedipine, a calcium channel blocker, may produce gingival hyperplasia.

The triad of hypertension, diabetes and oral lichenoid reaction has been termed 'Grinspan's syndrome', but in retrospect the lichenoid lesions described were probably secondary to antihypertensive or hypoglycaemic drug therapy and therefore the validity of the syndrome is questionable.

Angina

Patients with angina suffer a relative reduction in coronary artery bloodflow which leads to myocardial insufficiency. It is important to establish whether the patient's angina is stable (occurring after a known period of exercise) or unstable (occurring at any time including during routine dental treatment). Many patients with angina are prescribed glyceryl trinitrate, as a tablet or spray, to be taken sublingually during any acute attacks (fig. 11) and it is advisable to ensure that such patients have their medication with them when they attend the dental surgery. It has been claimed that anxious patients with an 'achiever' personality have an increased likelihood of developing angina. Therefore, it would seem prudent to arrange an early morning appointment for such patients to avoid them worrying about any prospective treatment all day.

Myocardial infarction

The occurrence of myocardial infarction (MI) or heart attack is associated with patients who are known to have hypertension, angina or high blood lipid levels. It has been recommended that routine dental treatment should, if possible, be avoided in the first 3 months after an MI and that no advanced or complex procedures should be undertaken for at least 12 months.

In order to reduce the risk of subsequent endocarditis, patients with valvular disorders of the heart as a result of rheumatic fever or surgery, require to be provided with antibiotic cover prior to dental procedures which may produce a bacteraemia. Although infective endocarditis is a rare disease it does carry a high mortality and therefore appropriate cover should be provided. It is currently recommended that patients should be given either 3 g of amoxycillin one hour pre-operatively (with an option of giving a second dose of 3 g, 6 hours later) or 1·5 g of erythromycin 1–2 hours pre-operatively with 0·5 g given 6 hours later. Amoxycillin is the drug of choice, whereas erythromycin can be used as an alternative for patients with a sensitivity to the penicillin group of antibiotics.

Respiratory disorders

Asthma and bronchitis are two of the commonest respiratory disorders in the UK. Treatment of patients with asthma often involves the use of steroid inhaler therapy, which can predispose to oral candidosis (figs 12 and 13). The likelihood of developing oral candidosis can be reduced if the patient is asked to rinse the mouth or gargle with water following the use of the inhaler. In severe cases of asthma, long-term systemic steroid therapy may be prescribed and as previously described there is a risk that this may produce adrenal suppression.

Neurological disorders

Epilepsy is a chronic disease characterised by transient episodes of central neuronal discharge. The clinical spectrum of epilepsy ranges from petit mal 'absences' to grand mal seizures. Although minor episodes are unlikely to cause any problems the patient may traumatise the oral mucosa, particularly the tongue, during a grand mal seizure (fig. 14). It has been suggested that a prop should be placed in the mouth of an epileptic patient during routine dental treatment, but this is unnecessary and in itself may be dangerous. It is also probably inadvisable to try to place a padded spatula between the teeth of a patient if a seizure does occur. However, the patient should be helped into the recovery position away from equipment and furniture. If the seizure persists then diazepam (10 mg) should be given slowly intravenously. In addition to the possibility of an epileptic seizure occurring in the dental surgery, epileptic patients receiving phenytoin therapy may also develop gingival hyperplasia (fig. 15). The hyperplasia seems to be partly related to poor oral hygiene and partly due to the ability of phenytoin to directly stimulate fibroblast proliferation.

Bleeding disorders

Bleeding disorders can be classified either as inherited or acquired. The inherited group includes haemophilia, Christmas disease and von Willebrand's disease. Patients with these disorders are registered at regional haemophiliac centres, from which information on the severity of their disease can be obtained. Regardless of the severity of the disease, it is probably best that these patients undergo any dental procedures which are likely to cause bleeding in a hospital setting, where appropriate supplements of clotting factors can be provided along with the antifibrinolytic drug tranexamic acid. Unfortunately, the inadvertent use of contaminated blood products in this group of patients has resulted in infection with hepatitis B virus and human immunodeficiency virus as a possible additional complication of their treatment.

Acquired bleeding disorders are usually either a direct result of coumarin anticoagulant therapy or a reduction in platelet levels (thrombocytopenia) caused by drugs or infection. Owing to the short life of platelets (8–12 days) and thus the likelihood of low levels becoming even lower, any patient suspected of having thrombocytopenia should be regarded as a medical emergency requiring immediate hospital referral. Patients receiving anticoagulant therapy may undergo routine or surgical dental treatment, although therapy should be appropriately monitored and adjusted by the patient's haematologist prior to any surgical procedures or tooth extraction.

Psychological problems

It has been reported that patients are more fearful of dental treatment than of major surgical operations and indeed the only condition feared more than receiving dental treatment is developing cancer. The severity of this fear is variable, but often manifests as a simple faint (syncope). Lying the patient down and elevating the legs to increase venous

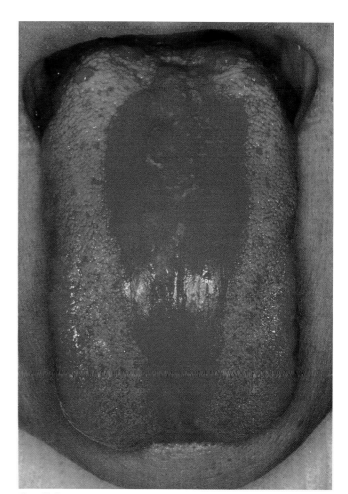

Fig. 12 Candidosis and papillary atrophy of the dorsum of the tongue in an asthmatic patient using steroid inhaler therapy.

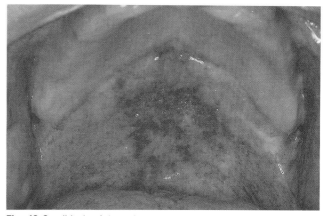

Fig. 13 Candidosis of the soft palate in a patient with severe asthma.

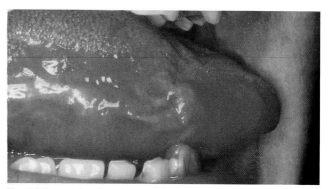

Fig. 14 Traumatic ulceration and hyperkeratosis of the tongue in a poorly controlled epileptic.

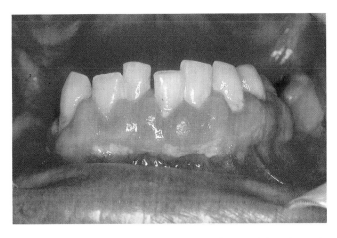

Fig. 15 Gingival hyperplasia in an epileptic patient receiving phenytoin therapy.

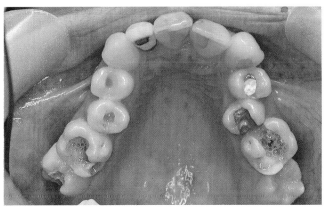

Fig. 16 This patient presented as shown. She had acute schizophrenia and had removed her amalgam restorations herself with a watchmaker's drill, in the belief that the metal in the fillings was acting as an 'aerial' for the reception of radio messages.

return to the heart will produce full recovery from a simple faint. However, if the bradycardia is sustained it may be necessary to give 0·2 mg of atropine subcutaneously or intramuscularly.

Acute anxiety may also produce alteration of acid-base balance by hyperventilation in which the patient complains of light-headedness, tingling in the extremities and tetany. Cases of hyperventilation are best treated by instructing the patient to breathe repeatedly into a plastic bag placed over the mouth and nose. The rationale for this is to allow the patient's carbon dioxide level to return to normal which will result in clinical recovery in around 5 minutes.

A caring and considerate approach by dental practitioners in an unhurried clinical setting with full explanation of proposed treatment can do much to allay patients' worries or fears. However, some patients remain frankly dental-phobic or needle-phobic and may require specialist help involving a clinical psychologist or hypnotherapy.

The dental practitioner should also be aware that patients can present with a variety of other psychological problems. Chronic anxiety can be an important component of burning mouth syndrome, whereas stress has been associated with the development of temporomandibular joint dysfunction, migraine on waking and recurrent aphthous stomatitis. Patients with a more profound psychological disorder, such as schizophrenia, may also present in dental practice with bizarre clinical findings (fig. 16). Obviously such patients require referral for appropriate treatment which can be organised through their general medical practitioner.

11
The immunocompromised patient

The immune system of a patient may be compromised, either owing to the presence of systemic disease or as a result of drug therapy. In this respect there can be no doubt that HIV infection and AIDS now dominate any discussion on the immunocompromised. The global significance of HIV infection is becoming increasingly apparent and is likely to have major implications for health care services well into the next century.

The emergence of HIV infection is likely to have a dramatic effect on the practice of dentistry. Although this chapter focuses on mucosal and infective disease associated with an immunocompromised state, other aspects of HIV infection, especially trigeminal neuralgia, trigeminal neuropathy, facial nerve palsy and dementia, should not be overlooked. The dental practitioner is uniquely trained to recognise oral disease, and it is application of this expertise, in conjunction with the medical practitioner, that will ensure appropriate health care of immunocompromised patients in the future.

Emergence of HIV infection

Human immunodeficiency virus (HIV), the agent now known to be responsible for AIDS, is a retrovirus which was initially called either LAV, HTLV-III or ARV. The immunodeficiency which characterises HIV infection develops as a result of a lymphotrophic and lymphocytopathic effect on T-helper lymphocytes. The first stage of infection involves attachment of the virus onto the lymphocytes by a specific antigen (T4). There is then a latent period, probably amounting to several years, during which the patient is an asymptomatic carrier prior to the development of clinical symptoms and, finally, full-blown AIDS. At the end of June 1991 in the UK, 15 712 individuals were known to be HIV-positive and 4758 patients had developed AIDS. The fatality of AIDS is expected to be close to 100% and, to date, approximately 50% of patients diagnosed as having AIDS have died.

Acquisition of HIV infection

It is now well recognised that HIV infection is transmitted by sexual intercourse, perinatally, by accidental blood contact or by provision of blood products. Unfortunately, many haemophiliacs, who depend on factor VIII derived from blood products, are now HIV-positive as a result of receiving untreated or unscreened blood factors. Saliva can also contain the HIV virus but at the present time the levels are regarded as being too low to be of clinical significance in terms of transmission of the disease. This consideration does not, however, in any way reduce the necessity for always wearing gloves in dental practice, not least because of the possibility of acquiring other viral infections, such as hepatitis B or herpes simplex.

Oral aspects of HIV infection

A significant proportion of research into HIV infection has focused on dental aspects, since it is becoming increasingly apparent that the oral cavity is a frequent site of clinical signs and symptoms of patients with HIV infection. The list of oral changes associated with HIV infection and AIDS continues to grow, but the most frequently seen lesions are oral candidosis (fig. 1), Kaposi's sarcoma (fig. 2), oral ulceration (fig. 3), non-Hodgkin's lymphoma (fig. 4), hairy leukoplakia

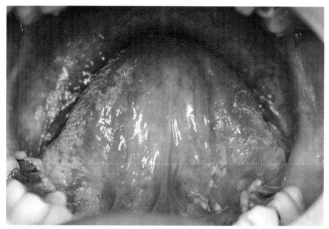
Fig. 1 Pseudomembranous candidosis of the floor of the mouth, ventral aspect of the tongue and retromolar area, in an AIDS patient.

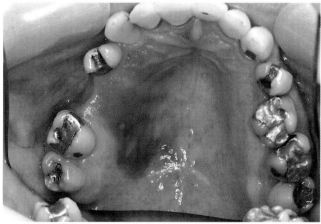
Fig. 2 Kaposi's sarcoma presenting with a typical bluish appearance, in an AIDS patient.

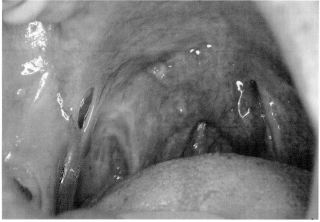
Fig. 3 Right tonsillar region showing large defect and scarring from a previous long-standing major aphthous type ulcer. Smaller areas of ulceration are also present.

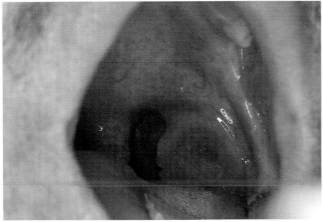

Fig. 4 Non-Hodgkin's lymphoma of the left tonsil was the only oral change in an AIDS patient.

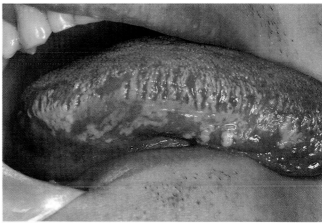

Fig. 5 Extensive hairy leukoplakia on the right lateral margin of the tongue.

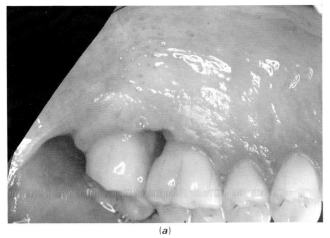

(a)

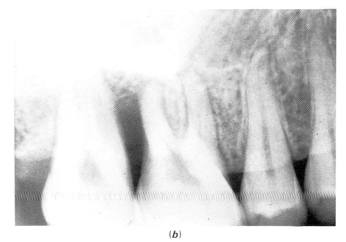

(b)

Fig. 6 (a) Clinical and (b) radiological appearance of rapidly progressing periodontitis in an AIDS patient.

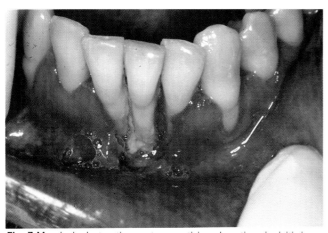

Fig. 7 Massively destructive acute necrotising ulcerative gingivitis in an HIV-positive patient.

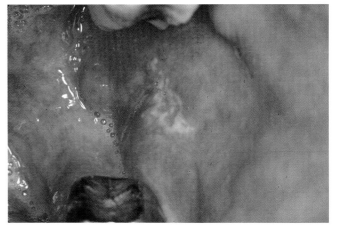

Fig. 8 Hairy leukoplakia of the buccal mucosa.

(fig. 5), rapidly progressive periodontitis (fig. 6) and acute necrotising ulcerative gingivitis (fig. 7). Other conditions which have been reported in HIV infection include herpes simplex infection, herpes zoster infection, papillomavirus lesions, xerostomia, parotitis, thrombocytopenia and squamous cell carcinoma.

The lesion of hairy leukoplakia was first described in San Francisco in 1984 and deserves special mention. Classically, this occurs bilaterally on the lateral margins of the tongue, but it is now known that it may develop at other mucosal sites such as the buccal mucosa (fig. 8) and labial mucosa. Although candidal infection co-exists in approximately half the cases of hairy leukoplakia, the lesion does not respond to antifungal therapy. *In situ* hybridisation studies of Epstein-Barr virus (EBV) has shown it to be an important factor in the development of hairy leukoplakia. Although hairy leukoplakia has a characteristic histopathological appearance, it is preferable to substantiate the clinical diagnosis by electron microscopy or DNA-hybridisation of EBV. Approximately 20% of patients with hairy leukoplakia have AIDS by the time they develop the lesion and, if they have not, the likelihood of developing AIDS in the next 2–5 years is around 80%. The diagnosis of hairy leukoplakia therefore has major prognostic significance in the development of AIDS. Factors such as the size of the lesion, clinical appearance or histological features do not correlate with the subsequent development of AIDS. Until recently, hairy leukoplakia was thought to be a pathognomic feature of HIV infection, but it is now apparent that it can occur in other immunocompromised patients, in particular those who have undergone renal transplantation. At the present time, acyclovir, in doses up to 2200 mg daily for 3 weeks, appears to be beneficial, although recurrence may occur following cessation of therapy.

Oral candidosis has been a recognised feature of AIDS since the original descriptions of the disease in 1981. Clinically, pseudomembranous (fig. 9) or erythematous forms of candidosis are predominant, although candida-associated angular cheilitis and median rhomboid glossitis have also been described.

Haemopoietic and lymphoreticular disease

Disorders of the haemopoietic and lymphoreticular systems result in a degree of immunocompromised states in the host. The most important of these disorders are those which affect the white blood cell series, either owing to a reduction in total number of cells (neutropenia or agranulocytosis) or to increase in numbers of cells, but with altered function (leukaemia).

Neutropenia

Neutropenia can be idiopathic or may occur as a result of drug therapy or marrow replacement by neoplastic tissue or myelofibrosis. The major oral sign of neutropenia is ulceration (fig. 10), which has been termed neutropenic ulceration since the ulcers seem to occur as a direct result of low white cell numbers. Such ulceration is difficult to treat but, following liaison with the patient's haematologist, drugs such as prednisolone or azathioprine have been found to be helpful (fig. 11). Mucosal infections are an additional problem of neutropenia and may be caused by *Varicella zoster* (fig. 12) or *Herpes simplex* virus, either intra-orally (fig. 13) or extra-orally (fig. 14).

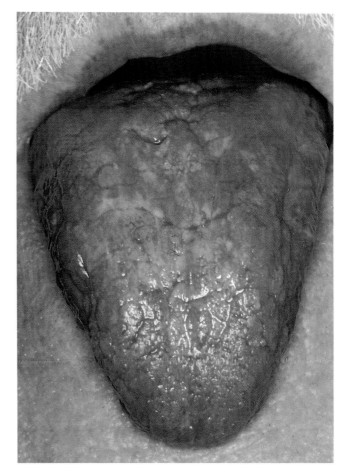

Fig. 9 Pseudomembranous candidosis with erythematous areas in an AIDS patient.

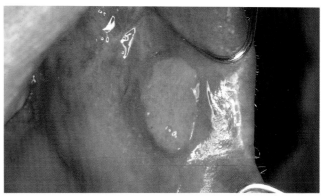

Fig. 10 Neutropenic ulceration in a patient with the myelodysplastic syndrome.

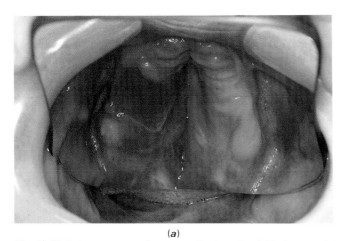
(a)

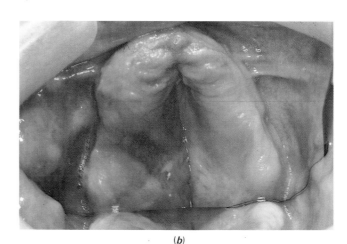
(b)

Fig. 11 Clinical appearance of neutropenic ulceration (a) before and (b) after 2 weeks of therapy with prednisolone and azathioprine.

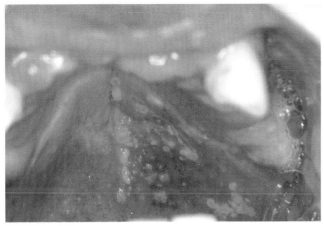

Fig. 12 *Herpes zoster* of the soft palate in a patient with neutropenia.

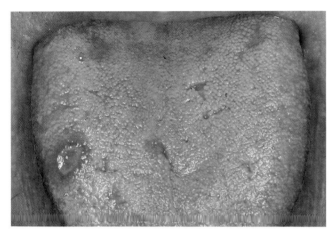

Fig. 13 *Herpes simplex* virus was isolated from this painful ulcer in a patient with neutropenia.

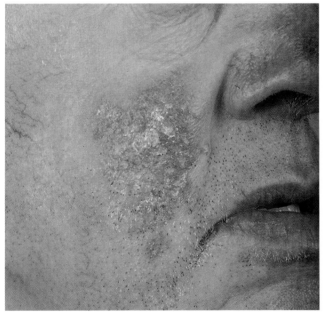

Fig. 14 Cutaneous *Herpes simplex* infection.

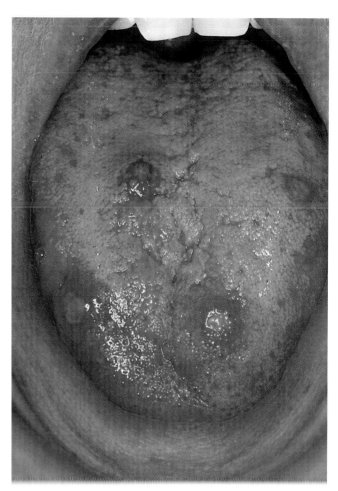

Fig. 15 *Herpes simplex* virus infection of the dorsum of the tongue in a patient with chronic lymphatic leukaemia.

Leukaemia

Gingival enlargement and bleeding are well recognised features of the acute leukaemias. Histological examination of gingival tissue from acute leukaemias reveals large numbers of white blood cells, reflecting the fact that although there is an increase in white cell numbers those that are present are functionally impaired. Oral ulceration, petechiae, viral infections and candidal infections (fig. 15) can all occur in patients with leukaemia. Since other cells derived from the marrow, such as platelets, are often reduced in numbers, these patients are also likely to have bleeding problems. The dentist has a significant role to play in the oral care of leukaemic patients and can do much to relieve oral discomfort, which is frequently a major complaint. Although patients with leukaemia are often prescribed prophylactic acyclovir, some are not and the dentist should be aware that any area of painful oral ulceration could possibly be of viral origin (fig. 15). In addition, since oral changes can occur early in the disease, suspicion of underlying disease warrants immediate referral to the patient's medical practitioner.

12

Special investigations

A variety of special investigations are routinely used to aid clinical diagnosis. Questions which need to be answered prior to the performance of any special investigation include: 'which tests are appropriate?', 'how should the specimen be obtained?' and 'how should the results be interpreted clinically?' It is clearly not necessary to perform a large number of special investigations on every patient and tests should therefore be limited to those which are most appropriate.

Improved understanding of human disease has led to the recognition that changes within the orofacial tissues can be the first indication of a number of systemic diseases. Therefore, the performance and interpretation of special investigations is likely to be increasingly important in the management of a dental patient. Liaison with the patient's doctor will increase the likelihood of early detection of disease and enhance the role of medical and dental practitioners as partners in the provision of health care. In this chapter it is proposed to discuss the investigations which are most frequently undertaken in oral medicine and to illustrate their relevance with examples of clinical conditions.

Venepuncture

Many investigations are based on analysis of blood (Tables I and II) and the clinician should therefore be adept at venepuncture. If a general dental practitioner wishes to perform venepuncture, then local hospitals are usually happy to supply appropriate needles, syringes, request forms and specimen bottles. In addition, the laboratory staff can be very helpful in advising on how best to perform a particular investigation and how they would prefer to receive the specimen. Alternatively, the patient's medical practitioner or local oral medicine consultant service can be asked to obtain any necessary samples.

Venepuncture is a straightforward procedure and the veins in the antecubital fossa (fig. 1) are the vessels of choice, owing to their adequate size and easy accessibility. Tourniquets are available, either in three predetermined sizes (small, medium or large) or in a universal format which is variable in length. It is important to choose a tourniquet that will be able to apply adequate pressure without being overtight. A syringe capable of containing the volume of blood required should be selected, along with an appropriate needle or butterfly. Needles and butterflies are colour-coded to indicate their internal diameter: blue (small) 23 gauge, green (medium) 21 gauge and white (large) 19 gauge (fig. 2). For most situations, the bore of a blue needle is too small to allow an adequate sample to be taken without the blood clotting. Although clotting is not a problem with the large white needles, their usefulness is limited since patients often find their insertion painful. A green needle (or butterfly) attached in such a way that the calibration on the syringe and the bevel of the needle both face the operator is therefore the best choice.

The clinician should wear gloves throughout the venepuncture and should only remove them once the specimen has been placed in appropriate bottles. The chosen tourniquet should be placed half way between the elbow and shoulder and the skin overlying the chosen vein swabbed with alcohol (fig. 3). The needle should be inserted at a 60° angle

Table I Special investigations		
Test	Sample	Comment
Haematology		
Full blood count	Pink top EDTA bottle 5 ml	Invert bottle 2-3 times after filling.
Corrected whole blood folate	Pink top EDTA bottle 5 ml	Invert bottle 2-3 times after filling.
Vitamin B12	White top plain tube 10 ml	
Ferritin	White top plain tube 10 ml	Preferable to serum iron and total iron binding capacity
Erythrocyte sedimentation rate	Purple Westergren bottle	Send to laboratory immediately
Clotting screen	Variable	Check with laboratory
Biochemistry		
Glucose (a) Random	Yellow top fluoride bottle 2·5 ml	Patient fasted overnight prior to collection
(b) Tolerance test	Yellow top fluoride bottle 2·5 ml	Two samples: Initial fasted then second sample 2 hours after oral administration of 75 g glucose
Alkaline phosphatase Gammaglutamyl transpeptidase Transaminase alanine	White top plain tube 10 ml	
Calcium Phosphate Urea Sodium Potassium Chloride	White top plain 10 ml	Calcium levels should be acquired with tourniquet off.
Cortisol (a) Random		Collect at 0.800-0.900 hours
(b) Synacthen test	White top plain 10 ml	Two samples; initial as random 0.800-0.900 hours Second sample 30 minutes after IV or IM administration of 0·25 mg tetracosactrin (synacthen).
Growth hormone	White top plain 10 ml	Send sample along with glucose tolerance test
Tri-iodothyronine (T3) Thyroxine (T4) Free thyroxine index (FTI)	White top plain 20 ml sample	Plastic or glass container—check with laboratory.

Table II Special immunological investigations

Test	Sample	Comment
Antinuclear antibody and rheumatoid factor	White top plain 10 ml	Positive in connective tissue disorders
Immunoglobulins IgG IgA IgM IgE	White top plain 10 ml	?Paraproteinaemia
IgE (RAST)	White top plain 10 ml	?Food or environmental allergens
Indirect immunofluorescence	White top plain 10 ml	?Vesiculobullous disease

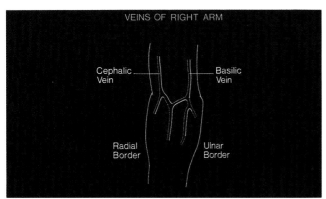

Fig. 1 Diagram of veins in the antecubital fossa.

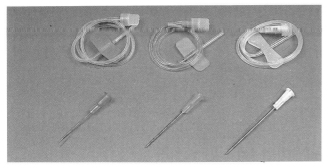

Fig. 2 Commonly available needles and butterflies. (The sterile packaging and needle covers have been removed for clarity.)

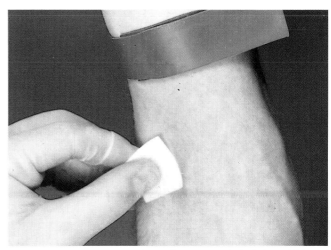

Fig. 3 Tourniquet positioned on the arm and alcohol swabbing of venepuncture site.

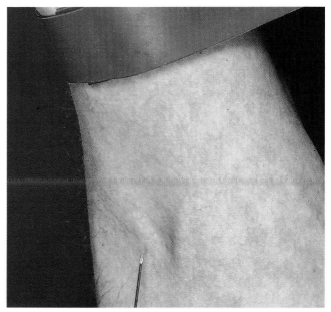

Fig. 4 Insertion of needle into vein.

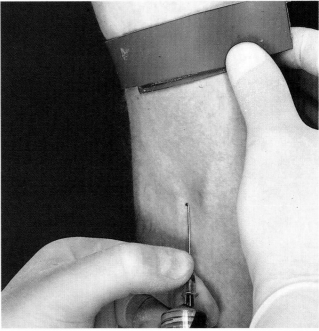

Fig. 5 Release of tourniquet immediately prior to removal of needle.

directly into the vein (fig. 4) and the index finger of the hand holding the syringe should be placed firmly against the skin to prevent withdrawal of the needle when aspiration of blood begins. Once the required volume of blood has been collected, the tourniquet should be released prior to removal of the needle (fig. 6). A gauze swab is then placed over the puncture site as the needle is withdrawn and the patient asked to hold this firmly in position. Some clinicians recommend that the patient should bend or elevate the arm at this stage to reduce the risk of bruising, but this is unnecessary and, in fact, is more likely to encourage bruising at the site of venepuncture. The needle should be removed from the syringe prior to filling the appropriate specimen bottles to the correct level. Each sample bottle should then be capped and those containing anticoagulant gently inverted two or three times. The needle and syringe should then be disposed of safely in a 'sharps' container. Finally, the patient's puncture site should be inspected and covered with an elastoplast provided the patient has no history of allergy to this type of dressing.

Specimen forms must be completed in full and bottles clearly labelled prior to transfer to the laboratory for processing. In routine cases, the patient is then reappointed 2–3 weeks later (depending on the type of tests which have been undertaken) to be informed of their results. However, in emergency situations, samples must be rapidly transported to the laboratory and arrangements made to contact the patient later the same day. Emergency conditions which may present at the general dental practice include thrombocytopenia, aplastic anaemia or acute leukaemia, all of which can produce oral lesions (figs 6 and 7).

Haematology

The haematological tests routinely carried out in oral medicine specialist clinics consist of a full blood count (FBC) and assays of levels of vitamin B12, ferritin (or iron/total iron binding capacity) and corrected whole blood folate (fig. 8). It is felt that the performance of these tests is justified in the initial management of aphthous ulceration and angular cheilitis, since haematological abnormalities occur in a significant proportion of patients with these conditions. In addition, they should be performed routinely in patients with atrophic glossitis, burning mouth syndrome or an unusually severe or prolonged oral infection.

Other haematological tests which may help in certain situations include erythrocyte sedimentation rate (ESR) in suspected cases of giant cell arteritis or systemic lupus erythematosus and coagulation studies in patients with possible bleeding disorders.

Biochemistry

The range of biochemical investigations now available is vast, but only a few, namely venous plasma blood glucose, gammaglutamyl transpeptidase (Gamma GT), aspartate transaminase (AST), alanine transaminase (ALT), alkaline phosphatase, serum calcium, serum phosphate, urea and electrolytes are commonly used in the practice of oral medicine. Occasionally, assays of hormones, such as cortisol, growth hormone, tri-iodothyronine (T3), thyroxine (T4) and free thyroxine index may also be helpful. Individual centres differ in the type of sample they require for these tests, but local preferences can be assessed by contacting the appropriate laboratory.

Routine measurement of venous plasma blood glucose in the management of burning mouth syndrome has revealed that approximately 1 in 20 of such patients are undiagnosed maturity onset diabetics. In addition, undiagnosed or poorly controlled diabetes mellitus has been implicated in a variety of other orofacial complaints, including candidosis, altered taste, sialosis and periodontal disease.

Elevated levels of liver enzymes (Gamma GT, AST and ALT) possibly with an increase in the mean corpuscular volume, would support the presence of alcohol abuse in a patient. Alcohol abuse has also been suggested as a cause of sialosis and has a well recognised association with the development of epithelial dysplasia and oral cancer. It is advisable to assess baseline levels of liver enzymes prior to prescribing either carbamazepine or griseofulvin, since these drugs can produce hepatic changes.

Pathological disorders involving changes in bone metabolism such as primary hyperparathyroidism, Paget's disease and fibrous dysplasia can all produce an increased level of alkaline phosphatase, although this enzyme will also be raised

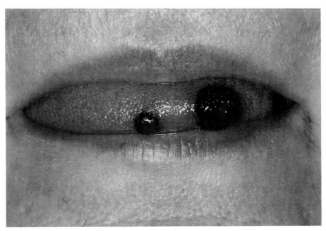

Fig. 6 Purpuric lesions of the tongue in thrombocytopenia.

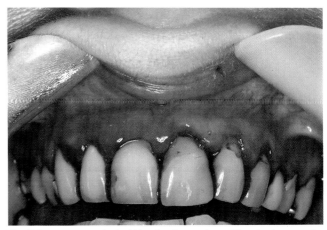

Fig. 7 Spontaneous gingival bleeding in a patient with aplastic anaemia.

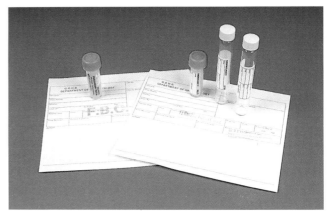

Fig. 8 Blood bottles and forms for haematological evaluation (FBC, corrected whole blood folate, ferritin and serum B12).

as a physiological growth response in children and adolescents. Levels of calcium and phosphate can be either elevated or reduced in some forms of hyperparathyroidism.

The adrenocortical dysfunction of Addison's disease, which is fatal if undiagnosed, should be suspected if a patient presents in the dental surgery with a complaint of increased mucosal and skin pigmentation. The presence of Addison's disease is supported by raised potassium and hypotension, but diagnosis should be confirmed by measurement of cortisol levels in the morning (8 am–9 am) and during a synacthen test.

Excessive production of growth hormone in acromegaly produces a characteristic orofacial appearance, involving a Class III malocclusion and spacing of the teeth (fig. 9).

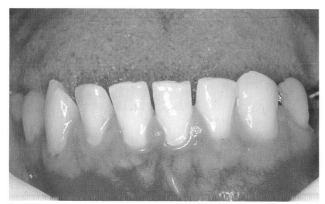

Fig. 9 Acromegaly presenting as spacing of the lower incisor teeth and a scalloped appearance to the lateral margin of the tongue. (Reprinted by kind permission from *Pocket picture guide: oral medicine.* London: Gower Medical Publishing, 1988.)

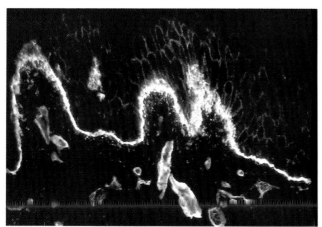

Fig. 10 Immunofluorescence demonstrating IgG along the basement membrane zone in a patient with pemphigoid (skin biopsy).

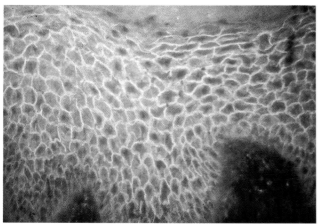

Fig. 11 Immunofluorescence demonstrating intercellular deposits of IgG in a patient with pemphigus (oral mucosa).

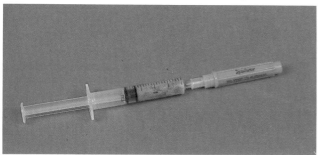

Fig. 12 Aspirate of pus.

Thyroid disorders are common and general dental practitioners can be the first to note the early signs of disease such as a malar flush in hypothyroidism and exophthalmos in hyperthyroidism. Confirmation of the clinical diagnosis is made by blood investigations involving measurement of levels of T3, T4 and free thyroxine index.

Immunology

Although general dental practitioners are unlikely to undertake immunological investigations for their patients, it is useful to be aware of the spectrum of immunological tests which are now available. Assessment of antinuclear antibody and rheumatoid factor should be performed in patients with xerostomia, particularly if Sjögren's syndrome is suspected, since it can confirm the presence of a connective tissue disorder, in particular systemic lupus erythematosus or rheumatoid arthritis. A refinement of these tests involving detection of double or single strand antibodies to DNA is now available and this is useful in determining whether the onset of Sjögren's syndrome has been induced by a drug, such as the antihypertensive hydralazine.

Assessment of serum IgE levels are of value in identifying atopic patients, and a radioallergosorbent test (RAST) will give levels of IgE to common allergens, in particular house dust mite, pollen and dog epithelium. Significant levels of IgE to these and other factors are present in approximately 50% of the patients with orofacial granulomatosis.

Immunofluorescence (IF), a type of immunological test, is invaluable in diagnosing vesiculobullous disorders, in particular pemphigus and pemphigoid. If a vesiculobullous disorder is suspected, then a 10 ml clotted blood sample should be sent, with a mucosal biopsy (on ice) for examination using direct and indirect IF techniques (figs 10 and 11).

Microbiology

Whenever possible a pus sample should be obtained from any suppurative infection occurring in the orofacial region. An aspirate (fig. 12) is far preferable to a swab since aspiration is much less likely to be associated with specimen contamination from the commensal oral microflora. Regardless of the method of sampling used, any specimen of pus obtained should be sent to the laboratory promptly. Any delay in transit will result in loss of viable organisms, especially oxygen-sensitive strict anaerobes.

The taking of smears is a convenient and rapid method of providing information on the likely identity of organisms present in an infection. This type of investigation is particularly helpful in demonstrating the fusobacteria/spirochaetal complex of acute necrotising ulcerative gingivitis (fig. 13) or determining whether lesions of angular cheilitis are due to infection with candida (fig. 14), staphylococci or a mixture of both types of organism.

In addition to smears, swabs should be taken from lesional sites and dentures (if worn) of any patient with a suspected oral candidosis. However, it is essential that swabs are not taken from any area of lesional mucosa which is subsequently to be biopsied, since surface layers may be removed which can complicate subsequent histopathological interpretation of the tissues. An oral rinse should be performed (fig. 15) in suspected cases of oral candidosis, since it is the most convenient method of quantitatively assessing the candidal

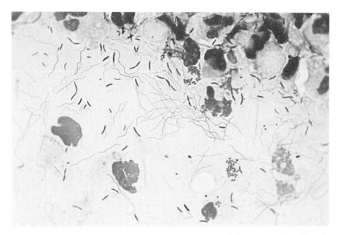

Fig. 13 Smear of acute necrotising ulcerative gingivitis stained by Gram's method, demonstrating numerous spirochaetes, fusobacteria and polymorphonuclear leucocytes.

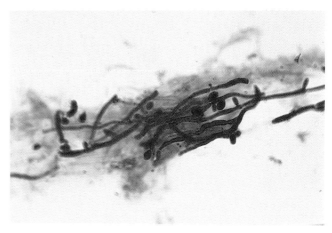

Fig. 14 Smear of angular cheilitis stained by Gram's method, demonstrating candidal species present in the blastospore and hyphal phases.

component of a patient's oral microflora.

Most viral infections encountered in general dental practice are due to the herpes group of viruses. Although diagnosis of primary herpetic gingivostomatitis can usually be made relatively easily from the characteristic clinical appearance, a swab of an oral ulcer should be taken and placed in virus transport medium (fig. 16) prior to transfer to the laboratory for confirmation of the presence of *Herpes simplex* virus.

The presence of virus is usually determined either by an immunofluorescent method or by demonstration of a cytopathic effect on cell culture lines (fig. 17). A blood sample taken in the acute phase of infection and again in the convalescent period (10–14 days later) should demonstrate at least a fourfold rise in antibody titre to *Herpes simplex* virus type I or II to confirm diagnosis. Laboratories do not routinely isolate *Varicella zoster* virus and therefore a clinical diagnosis of herpes zoster is usually confirmed by serological determination of antibody titres. Not only is it good practice to confirm suspected intra-oral viral infections by laboratory tests, it is also a useful way of obtaining good epidemiological data on the prevalence of disease.

The infectivity of individuals who have suffered viral hepatitis is determined haematologically and contact with the patient's general medical practitioner or regional virus laboratory will therefore usually reveal a patient's status. However, if there is doubt, an appropriately labelled serum sample should be sent to determine the presence of the following factors: HBsAg, anti-HBsAg, HBeAg, anti-HBeAg and DNA polymerase.

All members of the dental team should be vaccinated against hepatitis B virus and should subsequently be tested to ensure that they develop a significant level of antibody (seroconvertion). It is known that a small proportion of individuals who receive the hepatitis vaccine either do not seroconvert or develop only low levels of antibody. Antibody status should therefore be determined 3 months post-vaccination, and at regular intervals thereafter, since this will indicate the degree of protection and whether a further vaccination is required.

It is becoming increasingly apparent that acquired immunodeficiency syndrome (AIDS) may be first suspected from changes within the oral cavity. However, there is no justification for testing a patient's HIV status without their

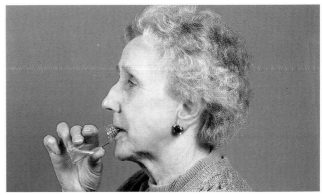

Fig. 15 Oral rinse technique. A 9 ml volume of phosphate-buffered saliva is held in the mouth for one minute prior to collection in a sterile container.

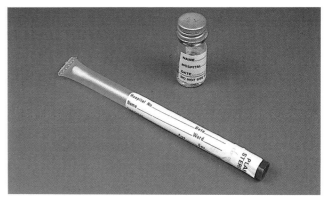

Fig. 16 Microbiological swab and viral transport medium.

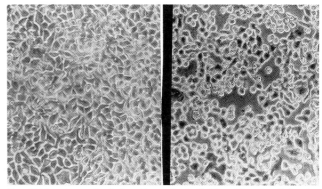

Fig. 17 Monolayer of cells in culture prior to (left) and five days following (right) inoculation with *Herpes simplex* virus.

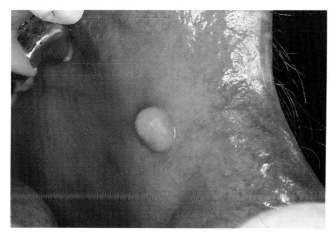

Fig. 18 Fibro-epithelial polyp.

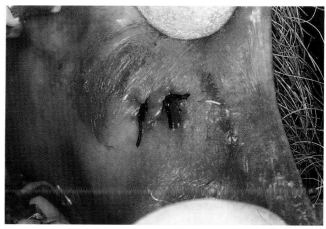

Fig. 19 Closure of mucosal biopsy site using interrupted black silk sutures.

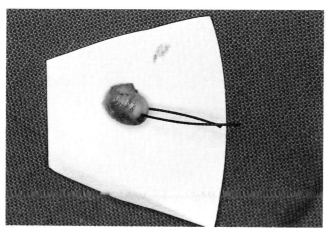

Fig. 20 Biopsy specimen with the epithelial surface uppermost placed on filter paper.

knowledge. Any patient suspected of being HIV-positive should initially be referred to a medical practitioner who will arrange professional counselling prior to any assessment.

Histopathology

Tissue biopsy is probably the most helpful investigation in determining mucosal disease. Opinions differ as to whether a biopsy of the oral mucosa should be performed by the patient's general practitioner or a specialist. Clearly, a simple benign localised lesion, such as a fibro-epithelial polyp, could be dealt with in the dental practice (figs 18 and 19), although it is essential to send all material removed for histopathological examination. However, many conditions have widespread mucosal involvement and it is the experience of knowing the area which is likely to provide the most useful information that is one of the main reasons that sampling is perhaps best performed in specialist centres. It is helpful to place biopsy material on a filter paper prior to immersion in formol saline (volume at least ten times that of the biopsy), since this prevents distortion of the biopsy during fixation (fig. 20).

Direct immunofluorescence is extremely useful in diagnosing bullous disorders and it is essential that biopsy material for this type of investigation is sent to the laboratory on ice. The taking of cytological smears can also be helpful in diagnosis of certain oral conditions, but the use of this type of test is limited owing to the danger of false negatives, particularly in the detection of dysplastic lesions within the mouth.

Sample transportation

It is essential that all specimens should be appropriately transported to the laboratory. A hospital or health centre is likely to have an established system for processing all types of specimens, but in a dental practice setting special arrangements will probably have to be made. If immediate transportation is not possible, then blood samples, apart from those for either full blood count or glucose, can be placed in the fridge overnight without detriment. There is no urgency to transport tissue biopsies which have been placed in formalin and special containers for sending such specimens through the post are widely available (fig. 21). If samples are sent through the post, then there are strict requirements from the Post Office; these include the use of padded containers to absorb any fluid in the event of leakage and labelling to indicate the presence of a pathological specimen.

Interpretation of laboratory data

Interpretation of results of any special investigation is influenced by the sex and age of the patient and the presence of any known medical condition or drug history. With regard to blood investigations, it is also important to know the units and normal range used by the laboratory which performed the test. If the laboratory report states that the specimen was unsuitable for analysis or incomplete clinical details were provided, then the test should be repeated.

Most blood assays of a haematological or biochemical

nature are sufficiently accurate and reliable for appropriate treatment to be instituted on the basis of initial results. One possible exception to this is the situation where a marginally low vitamin B12 level is accompanied by a normal mean corpuscular volume. Under these circumstances the B12 assay should be repeated to determine if a deficiency truly exists and therefore if further investigation is indicated. The dental surgeon should bring the detection of any abnormal result to the attention of the patient's general medical practitioner since it is likely to have implications for further management. A common example of this is the detection of iron deficiency since this is not a disease in itself but reflects factors of either inadequate intake, malabsorption or excessive loss, all of which require investigation prior to the institution of any replacement therapy.

Interpretation of the results of bacterial or fungal investigations is usually straightforward since the report will provide identity and antimicrobial sensitivity of any microorganisms isolated. On the basis of this information antimicrobial chemotherapy can either be instituted or changed as necessary if clinical improvement has not occurred to any empirical treatment. Results of virological and immunological tests can also be interpreted relatively easily.

Although the majority of histopathological reports give a definitive diagnosis, occasions do arise when the information provided is equivocal. In such cases it is preferable to send biopsy material to an oral pathologist rather than a general pathology department.

Summary
Diagnostic services provide a valuable aid to patient management and consultants in charge of laboratories are

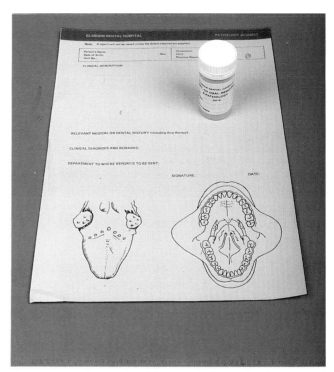

Fig. 21 Request form and container suitable for sending formalin-fixed tissues by post.

usually very willing to provide helpful information to the clinician on how best to proceed with investigations. Hopefully, in the future, much closer links will be established between dentistry and medicine as partners in the provision of patient health care. One way in which these links could be established is the performance or arrangement of appropriate specimen investigations within general dental practice.

Index